Pediatric Mental and Behavioral Health in Practice

A Case-Based Guide

Katie Lockwood, MD, MEd, FAAP
Billie Schwartz Abraham, PhD

American Academy of Pediatrics
DEDICATED TO THE HEALTH OF ALL CHILDREN®

American Academy of Pediatrics Publishing Staff
Jeff Mahony, *Senior Director, Professional and Consumer Publishing*
Carrie Peters, *Editor, Professional/Clinical Publishing*
Shannan Martin, *Production Manager, Consumer Publications*
Amanda Helmholz, *Medical Copy Editor*
Soraya Alem, *Manager, Digital Publishing*
Sara Hoerdeman, *Marketing and Acquisitions Manager, Consumer Products*

Published by the American Academy of Pediatrics
345 Park Blvd
Itasca, IL 60143
630/626-6000
www.aap.org

The American Academy of Pediatrics is an organization of 67,000 primary care pediatricians, pediatric medical subspecialists, and pediatric surgical specialists dedicated to the health, safety, and well-being of all infants, children, adolescents, and young adults.

While every effort has been made to ensure the accuracy of this publication, the American Academy of Pediatrics does not guarantee that it is accurate, complete, or without error.

The recommendations in this publication do not indicate an exclusive course of treatment or serve as a standard of medical care. Variations, taking into account individual circumstances, may be appropriate.

Statements and opinions expressed are those of the authors and not necessarily those of the American Academy of Pediatrics.

Any websites, brand names, products, or manufacturers are mentioned for informational and identification purposes only and do not imply an endorsement by the American Academy of Pediatrics (AAP). The AAP is not responsible for the content of external resources. Information was current at the time of publication.

The publishers have made every effort to trace the copyright holders for borrowed materials. If they have inadvertently overlooked any, they will be pleased to make the necessary arrangements at the first opportunity.

This publication has been developed by the American Academy of Pediatrics. The contributors are expert authorities in the field of pediatrics. No commercial involvement of any kind has been solicited or accepted in the development of the content of this publication. Financial and conflict of interest disclosures for the authors of this book can be found at https://publications.aap.org/aapbooks/pages/ma1252.

Every effort has been made to ensure that the drug selection and dosages set forth in this publication are in accordance with the current recommendations and practice at the time of publication. It is the responsibility of the health care professional to check the package insert of each drug for any change in indications or dosage and for added warnings and precautions.

Every effort is made to keep *Pediatric Mental and Behavioral Health in Practice: A Case-Based Guide* consistent with the most recent advice and information available from the American Academy of Pediatrics.

Please visit www.aap.org/errata for an up-to-date list of any applicable errata for this publication.

Special discounts are available for bulk purchases of this publication. Email Special Sales at nationalaccounts@aap.org for more information.

Printed in the United States of America

9-539 1 2 3 4 5 6 7 8 9 10

MA1252

ISBN: 978-1-61002-921-6

eBook: 978-1-61002-922-3

Cover and publication design by Peg Mulcahy

Library of Congress Control Number: 2026935888

American Academy of Pediatrics Reviewers

Committee on Drugs

Committee on Psychosocial Aspects of Child and Family Health

Committee on Substance Use and Prevention

Council on Adolescents and Young Adults

Council on Community Pediatrics

Council on Early Childhood

Council on School Health

National Center for Relational Health and Trauma-Informed Care Expert Leadership Team

Section on Clinical Pharmacology and Therapeutics

Section on Developmental and Behavioral Pediatrics

Authors

Katie Lockwood, MD, MEd, FAAP, is an attending physician at Children's Hospital of Philadelphia (CHOP) and works in primary care in Flourtown, PA. She is an associate professor of pediatrics at the University of Pennsylvania Perelman School of Medicine and holds a Distinguished Endowed Chair in the Department of Pediatrics as the director of behavioral health education in the CHOP Pediatric Residency Program. She is the creator and host of a podcast for pediatricians, *Primary Care Perspectives*.

Billie Schwartz Abraham, PhD, is a pediatric psychologist in private practice in California. Before this position, she was an assistant professor of clinical psychiatry at the University of Pennsylvania Perelman School of Medicine and a clinical psychologist at the Children's Hospital of Philadelphia for 10 years. Her clinical and research focus was on integrated behavioral health in pediatric primary care and urban community settings.

Contents

Preface

There's one patient who changed how I would see every patient after. If I had to give her a pseudonym for this book, it would be Sunshine—not only because her personality was sunny but also because caring for her shone a light on the importance of mental health in pediatric care and changed the type of pediatrician I would become.

Sunshine had a chronic disease that was slowly killing her, and unfortunately she knew it. Her baseline sunny disposition as she greeted us on rounds, with tales of her scintillating adolescent life, fizzled out as her hospital admissions racked up. As her medical team, we thought we could make her happier by offering her hope in the form of scientific breakthroughs: A new drug! A transplant! Try this new device! As we worked harder and harder to manage her illness, she took matters into her own hands, in the form of substance misuse, to manage her pain. When I was a third-year pediatric resident, she died of a drug overdose, and while we will never know if it was unintentional or intentional, what struck me most was that maybe it was preventable.

Sunshine showed me that we were not treating a whole person when we focused on her chronic disease alone or when her therapists focused solely on her mental health. She was not a person with a disease and depression, as her case was much more nuanced and bidirectional: she was a person whose disease caused depression, or maybe brought it to light, and, in turn, her depression worsened her disease management. It was all interwoven, so I often wonder how her story would have been different if all her pediatric clinicians had been better trained in mental health care and her therapists had been integrated into her medical team.

Every time I have patients who are struggling with depression or suicidality, I think of Sunshine and what she would want me to do for them. I tell their caregivers that these are the children whose cases keep me up at night. They are the children to whom I wish I could give a glimpse into their future, showing them that their circumstances can get better. They need the adults in their life to work together. These are the children for whom Sunshine came into my life, so I could help.

In 2018, my hospital started to integrate behavioral health professionals such as psychologists, psychiatrists, and clinical social workers into some primary care practices. This is where I met Dr Schwartz Abraham, who is a clinical psychologist specializing in pediatric primary care psychology. This level of integration has been a game changer, not only for our patients but also for all the health care professionals and trainees who now get to learn from each other, practice at the top of their licenses, and work as an integrated team to better care for patients.

Each case in this book is an amalgamation of cases of the many children and families that Dr Schwartz Abraham and I have cared for over the years, both as individuals and as an integrated team. None of the cases in this book are derived directly from any one patient, and any similarity to an individual's case is merely a coincidence. Rather, they are a merger of many children's cases that have shaped both our careers. They involve the complex presentations that benefit most from integrated team management. The children in these cases challenge us to be better clinicians and inspire us to keep learning more. They are our greatest teachers. And, like Sunshine, they have made an impact on us.

We thought of each of these cases as a force of nature all their own. So we assigned the cases nature archetypes. Each chapter revolves around the theme of the archetype, not only the medical or behavioral diagnosis. The archetypes respect that our patients rarely come to the office with one concern or issue but rather come with complex, nuanced, and evolving cases, such as the natural elements after which these cases have been named. Embarking on any nature expedition can be overwhelming, but we hope you will turn to this book often as a resource in navigating mental health care. We aim for this book to be a guide to finding these children in the wilds of your pediatric practice.

And, most of all, we hope that when you see Sunshine in your clinic or hospital, you can help her because you have heard her story here.

Acknowledgments

To my patients: Thank you for your honesty and bravery in sharing your mental/behavioral health concerns with me. I am honored to be your pediatrician.

In 2020, I took on the role of director of behavioral health education for the Pediatric Residency Program at Children's Hospital of Philadelphia (CHOP). CHOP invested in this curriculum before the Accreditation Council for Graduate Medical Education made it a requirement thanks to the leadership of Drs Dan West, Joe St. Geme, Tami Benton, Beth Rezet, and Nathan Blum. I learned alongside our residents from my talented associate directors, Drs Katrina Fletcher and Alyssa Rosen.

One day at a conference, 2 mentors told me I should write a book. Fortunately, I agreed with them and so did AAP Publishing. Thank you for the nudge and believing in me, Drs Ken Ginsburg and Paul Offit.

Thank you to the early readers, who helped share their expertise to make this book better: Rachel Cohen and Drs Sam Neher, Andrew Grossman, Christina Holbein, and Katrina Fletcher.

Innumerable thanks to anyone who identifies as the Cluster, Goofy Little Skillet, or CHOP/South Philly/Flourtown—your support means everything.

To my coauthor, Billie: You know that from the second I first saw you, I knew we would be friends. I also knew you would break my heart when you moved away, and you did, but we're making long-distance friendship work. We wrote a book!

To my family: Lori, Gary, Bill, Susan, Steve, Jia, Tommy, Ally, Dylan, and Kelly, as well as Moira, Pat, and Matt, thank you for supporting and loving me, especially on the arduous journey to becoming a pediatrician.

To my husband, Brian, who grounds me, makes me laugh, goes along with my adventures, and stops me from joining more committees: I will always love you. Thank you for being the rock of our family; without you, none of this is possible.

To my children, Noah and Gwen: I hope you always feel my fierce love for you and know it is unwavering and unconditional. You are my greatest teachers, and you make me want to be my best self. My passions and career are focused on improving the lives of children, including, most of all, yours.

—KL

Bridging the gap between mental health and pediatric health care is more than a professional interest for me—it is my true passion. Throughout my journey, I have been fortunate to receive an abundance of support and guidance from mentors who have played a pivotal role in shaping both my approach to patient care and my training as a clinician.

To my CHOP family in Healthy Minds, Healthy Kids and in the South Philadelphia Care Network, I extend my deepest gratitude. You have provided me with an enriching clinical environment and a dynamic academic network, enabling me to deliver high-quality patient care, engage in collaborative research, and participate in meaningful training within this setting. I am especially thankful to my mentors, Drs Jennifer Matone, Paul Robbins, and Tom Power. Each of you has demonstrated what it means to be an academic clinician in pediatric primary care. I will always appreciate that you took a chance on me as a trainee, supported my professional growth, and helped shape me into the person and clinician I am today. Jen, your unwavering support since 2013 has meant everything to me. I would not have been able to write a book like this without your steadfast guidance, encouragement, and, above all, friendship. Last, a big thank-you to all my patients and families—your trust in me is the greatest honor.

To my family, thank you for your incredible support and belief in me. To my husband, Dan, your unwavering support and unconditional love have been my anchor. I am truly fortunate to have you as my partner in life, and I could not have achieved this without you by my side. To my children, Benjamin and Zachary, you are the greatest joys of my life. Every day, you inspire me and teach me how to be a better psychologist, teacher, and parent.

Katie, this journey began over coffee many years ago when we first dreamed up this idea. Despite your initial impression that I might be a transient psychologist who would not remain in your orbit, you took a chance on me. We not only built a strong professional relationship but also developed a wonderful friendship. I truly treasure our partnership, and I am so excited to continue this journey together. You are stuck with me now, so thank you most of all!

—BSA

Part I

Case Presentations

CHAPTER 1

Somatic Symptoms or Panic Disorder

Lightning: Characterized by episodic, intense sensations and feeling of impending doom.

Presentation

Sydney, a 16-year-old girl, has come to your office for her routine health supervision visit. She says she has been experiencing chest pain, which she describes as uncomfortable, and points to the location where she feels the pain (mid-sternum). She confirms the pain is not associated with exercise. She says that when she has the chest pain, she can feel palpitations and has nausea and dizziness. Her most recent episode happened when she was on her way to school this morning, and she explains that mornings are the most common time for these pain episodes. They have been happening more frequently in the past 2 weeks. Since the chest pain started, she has not been sleeping well at night and has missed a few days of school because of her pain. She is growing well, her physical examination findings are normal, and her visit is otherwise unremarkable.

In reviewing her health record, you note that she had supraventricular tachycardia (SVT) as an infant and was briefly taking propranolol. She was discharged by her cardiologist 5 years ago. Her most recent electrocardiogram report indicates "there is subtle evidence of ventricular preexcitation," but the record note states that her condition is stable and requires "no precautions/restrictions."

Patient History and Review of Systems

- **Birth history:** Full term, no complications.
- **Medical history:** SVT as an infant.
- **Family history:** Older brother with a leaky valve, grandma with heart problems.
- **Social history:** Lives at home with her mom and older brother. Her dad is in the military and currently deployed. She is in 11th grade and is an honor roll student. She responds that she does not use drugs, alcohol, or tobacco. She has not been sexually active. She sees her strengths as having a work ethic and being a good friend.
- **Medications:** None.
- **Constitutional:** No fevers, weight loss/gain, or night sweats.
- **HEENT:** No vision changes.
- **Respiratory:** No cough or shortness of breath.
- **Gastrointestinal:** No vomiting, diarrhea, or heartburn; positive for nausea.
- **Integumentary:** No rashes.
- **Lymphatic:** No enlarged lymph nodes.
- **Neurological:** No headaches; positive for dizziness.

➤ **What do you think is causing Sydney's chest pain?**

Differential Diagnosis

For an adolescent with chest pain, the differential diagnosis should include the following conditions:

- **Arrythmia:** Prior history of SVT; possible family history; symptoms of chest pain and palpitations.
- **Costochondritis**
  - — No known trigger reported, and pain not reproducible on exam.
  - — Also, this diagnosis does not explain the other symptoms of nausea and dizziness.
- **Asthma**
  - — Chest pain and shortness of breath are common asthma symptoms. The experience of an asthma flare, especially a first-time flare, can provoke anxiety.

  - Albuterol use can also cause tachycardia. In this case, there is no known prior history of asthma. Also, her symptoms are not provoked by exercise and are more common in the morning, which is atypical for asthma.
- **Gastroesophageal reflux:** Can present with substernal chest pain and nausea but should not cause dizziness or palpitations. Also, the patient's symptoms are not worse after eating, which makes reflux less likely.
- **Depression:** Poor sleep and acute change in school attendance could be signs of depression in an adolescent.
- **Panic disorder:** Recurring panic attacks, with 1 or more attacks followed by at least 1 month of fear of another panic attack or significant maladaptive behaviors related to the attacks.
- **Trauma:** Previous history of trauma exposure can produce symptoms that closely resemble anxiety or produce somatic symptoms such as unexplained chest pain.
- **Somatic symptom disorder:** There is a focus here on physical symptoms that is resulting in distress and interference with functioning.

Keep in Mind: Comorbidities

These diagnoses are not mutually exclusive; sometimes an organic etiology can exacerbate underlying anxiety or depression symptoms.

Additionally, because Sydney's chest pain may be caused by anxiety, refer to the *Diagnostic and Statistical Manual of Mental Disorders, Fifth Edition, Text Revision* (*DSM-5-TR*) for the classification of anxiety to see which description aligns with the patient's presentation.

- Generalized anxiety disorder[1]
  - Excessive anxiety and worry about several events or activities. Fears tend to be out of proportion to the situation/fear and significantly interfere with functioning. Anxiety examples include those around school or athletic performances, around public speaking, and around social/peer relationships.
- Panic disorder[2]
  - A recurrent unexpected, abrupt surge of intense fear or discomfort that reaches a peak within minutes and includes symptoms such as sweating, trembling, palpitations, and dizziness. The disorder occurs when multiple panic attacks occur, and anticipation of future attacks interferes with daily functioning.

- Social anxiety disorder[3]
  — Marked fear or anxiety about one or more social situations in which the individual is exposed to possible scrutiny by others. In children, the anxiety must occur in settings with peers and not just during interactions with adults.

Keep in Mind: Information Gathering

It can be helpful to ask the patient about the pattern of symptoms over time, beyond having them simply report their symptoms. Try to get an understanding of when these symptoms occur and if they interfere with the patient's daily life. With children, asking questions in a casual, conversation-like way may be most effective.

- Are the times of pain more common in the mornings, in the evenings, on weekdays, or during weekends? Do they happen more at school or home?
- Is anything happening right before or right after the pain starts/ends?
- Do they occur on summer break, holiday breaks, or event days at school (eg, theme days, field trips)?
- Have they ever interrupted a fun activity?

In this case, the somatic symptoms of chest pain, nausea, and dizziness, as well as the disruption of sleep and school attendance, combined with frequent worries about additional episodes of these symptoms, lead you to suspect that Sydney has an anxiety disorder.

➤ **What are the next steps to confirm the diagnosis?**

Evaluation

To evaluate a patient for an anxiety disorder, use a standardized psychosocial screening instrument. Many are in the public domain and do not require mental health training or scoring software; thus, they can be used in the pediatric clinical setting. For Sydney's evaluation, there are a few to consider. Refer to the Appendix for links to the tools online.

- **Screen for Child Anxiety Related Emotional Disorders (SCARED):** A pediatric anxiety screener used for children 8 years and older. A total score of 25 or higher may indicate the presence of an anxiety disorder. Child and parent rating scale versions are available.
  — Additionally, this screener will give the clinician subscale scores, which may indicate a specific type of anxiety disorder such as generalized anxiety disorder, social anxiety disorder, panic, school anxiety, and separation anxiety.

- **Generalized Anxiety Disorder-7 (GAD-7):** An efficient, 7-question self-report tool for youth aged 13 to 17 years for screening, diagnosis, and severity assessment of generalized anxiety disorder. The GAD-7 does not separate types of anxiety but provides a total score.
  - Cutoff scores are
    - 5–9—mild
    - 10–14—moderate
    - 15–21—severe
  - A score of 8 or higher is considered atypical and warrants further evaluation for the presence of an anxiety disorder.
- **Strengths and Difficulties Questionnaire (SDQ):** A general behavioral screening questionnaire, for children and adolescents aged 2 to 17 years, that focuses on emotional symptoms, conduct, hyperactivity/impulsivity, peer relationships, and prosocial behavioral concerns. The questionnaire does not follow diagnostic criteria as the former 2 questionnaires do but can flag areas of concern and prosocial strengths.
  - 25 items; can be completed by parents, teachers, or child (age dependent)
- **Patient Health Questionnaire-9 Modified for Adolescents (PHQ-A):** A depression and suicidality screening tool for youth aged 11 to 17 years. The PHQ-A consists of 8 items that help classify differences in levels of depressive symptoms and 1 item related to suicidal ideation (eg, "Thoughts that you would be better off dead, or of hurting yourself in some way?"). It can be a helpful tool when assessing for anxiety, as the 2 disorders are highly comorbid. It can also serve as a symptom tracker and progress-monitoring tool if used over time.
  - Cutoff scores are
    - 5—mild
    - 10—moderate
    - 15—moderately severe
    - 20—severe
  - If suicidal ideation is endorsed, it requires immediate follow-up with a more investigative suicide screener, such as the Ask Suicide-Screening Questions (ASQ) or Columbia-Suicide Severity Rating Scale (C-SSRS); safety planning; and referral for external support. Refer to Chapter 9, Suicidality and Eating Disorder, for further discussion on suicidality.
- **Pediatric Symptom Checklist-17 (PSC-17):** Widely used parent-completed measure of a child's psychosocial functioning, normed for children and adolescents aged 4 to 17 years, including internalized problems (eg, anxiety, depression), attention issues, and externalizing problems (eg, disruptive and oppositional behaviors). This is a briefer version of the PSC-35. Refer to Chapter 5, Somatic Symptoms and Depression, for additional details.
  - A score of 15 or higher suggests the need for further follow-up and an evaluation for the presence of a mental health disorder. Similarly, each subscale has a cutoff score.
    - Attention—7
    - Externalizing—7
    - Internalizing—5

To understand more about the history of the patient's symptoms, or the frequency in which they occur, consider asking the patient and/or caregiver some questions, such as

- Has there been anything upsetting or stressful that has happened recently?
- Have you (or has your child) experienced these chest pains before in your (their) life?
- Do you know if anyone in the family has had pains like this before?
- How are these symptoms affecting home, school, and social life?
- Do they get better if you (or your child) stay(s) home from school or during vacation/school breaks/school holidays?

Back to the Case

You decide to administer the SCARED to assess Sydney for an anxiety disorder. Based on her scores (Table 1-1), the length of time she has been experiencing symptoms, and the clinical interview, she meets criteria for an anxiety disorder, specifically panic disorder.

Table 1-1. Sydney's Scores on the SCARED

Anxiety Subscales	Positive Score	Patient Score
Generalized Anxiety Disorder	9	10
Separation Anxiety Disorder	5	4
Social Anxiety Disorder	8	5
Panic Disorder/Significant Somatic Symptoms	7	16
Significant School Avoidance	3	6
Total Score	*≥25*	*41*

Abbreviation: SCARED, Screen for Child Anxiety Related Emotional Disorders.

A diagnosis of panic disorder includes at least 4 weeks of panic-related symptoms, which may include palpitations, sweating, chest pain, nausea, and fear of losing control.[2]

➤ **Based on the information gathered so far during the visit, is any further medical evaluation needed for Sydney's somatic symptoms of chest pain?**

The decision to evaluate further for the potential cause of Sydney's chest pain may depend on your clinical suspicion. It is important to remember that medical and mental health evaluations can happen simultaneously, and findings from one do not exclude those from the other as a possible diagnosis. Certainly, Sydney's symptoms could be suggestive of sinus tachycardia or SVT, and given her history, you may want to explore this further. A 48-hour Holter monitor may help document an episode.

You recommend that Sydney see a cardiologist to ensure that SVT is not causing her symptoms. In the meantime, you ask her to limit her caffeine consumption and work on her sleep hygiene. Given that you are concerned she has panic disorder, and her symptoms have been interfering with sleep and school, you also recommend that she see a mental health specialist.

Brief interventions: While Sydney is awaiting an appointment with a mental health specialist, there are some brief interventions that can be introduced in the office setting. You can demonstrate quick relaxation skills and recommend resources for mindfulness, aromatherapy, meditation, and/or progressive relaxation.

- **Box breathing:** Inhale for 4 seconds, hold for 4, exhale for 4, and hold for 4.
- **Grounding:** 5-4-3-2-1 method—Identify 5 things you see, 4 things you feel, 3 things you hear, 2 things you smell, and 1 thing you taste.
- **Cognitive reframing:** "I am safe. This feeling will pass."

A month later, Sydney is cleared by the cardiologist and follows up with you. She reports that her symptoms are getting worse and now she is missing so much school that she is at risk of failing 11th grade. She says she can't concentrate at school because she's so tired. When you ask about her sleep, she says she wakes up a lot because of nightmares, but she can't remember what they are about.

In Sydney's case, we do not know of any trauma, but we should still use a trauma-informed care approach. Her nightmares and anxiety could be related to a prior trauma. You can let Sydney know that she can always talk with you about things that may feel scary or upsetting and that your job is to keep her safe.

Keep in Mind: Trauma-Informed Care

Most children will experience some type of trauma during childhood. Traumatic stress symptoms in children include reexperiencing (eg, imagery, nightmares), avoidance (eg, diminished interest, self-isolation, detachment), and hyperarousal (eg, anxiety, sleep disturbance, irritability, physical symptoms).

- The trauma-informed care (TIC) approach is the use of a framework to understand how traumatic events and subsequent experiences can have lasting effects on a person's health and wellness.[4] The goal of TIC is to move from asking "What's wrong with you?" to instead asking "What's happened to you?"
- TIC uses 5 guiding principles: safety, choice, collaboration, trustworthiness, and empowerment. It is not meant to be an afterthought in assessment or a questionnaire to complete but rather a framework or lens through which to view all patient care, regardless of whether trauma is known at the point of patient interaction.[5,6]

Socially, Sydney has stopped going out to eat with her friends because she's worried about having a panic attack. She also says she has a fear of choking and, because of that, often skips meals. Her friends and family are worried that she is losing weight. She continues to have episodes of chest pain, nausea, and dizziness. Sydney says she does not understand how her anxiety is causing physical symptoms in her body.

- You can explain the mind-body connection. When our brain senses a threat, it activates a fight-or-flight reaction. Think about our ancestors, who may have been out looking for food and come face-to-face with a lion. If there was a lion standing there in front of you, your body would prepare to either fight the lion or run away (flight).
  — For this reaction, your body needs to do several things[7]: increase heart rate to pump blood faster, increase respiratory rate to oxygenate that blood, dilate pupils so you can see better, tense up muscles, and release waste (stool and urine).
- All these responses in the body come from the brain when it sees a threat. They make sense when you are staring at a lion, but they also happen when your brain senses something that worries you, or a fear. What we need to do is help the brain understand that the worry or fear is not a real lion. We need to teach it *not* to activate the fight-or-flight reaction to things that are not real dangers.
- This is how the mind-body connection works in anxiety and anxiety treatment.

••• Communication Pearl ••• Obtaining Context

It's important to think about context and emotions when asking about any mental health concerns. Consider asking the patient

- Can you describe how you feel when I say the word *anxiety*?
- Would you agree that you feel stressed or anxious?
- How are these symptoms of anxiety interfering with your ability to function in your day-to-day life?
- When you feel this way, who do you talk with or what do you do to help yourself feel better?
- Would you like to be connected to a specialist who can help you manage these feelings so they don't have to get in the way of your life?

Discussion

Remember that anxiety can be comorbid with other diagnoses and managing/treating anxiety does not mean clinicians should not also entertain other possible explanations simultaneously.

- Common coexisting conditions with anxiety include
  - Attention-deficit/hyperactivity disorder
  - Autism spectrum disorder
  - Bullying
  - Depression
  - Eating disorders
  - Learning disability
  - Pregnancy
  - Substance use disorder
- Consider medical diagnoses that may coexist with anxiety or mimic anxiety symptoms, such as
  - Arrhythmias
  - Asthma
  - Food allergies
  - Hyperthyroidism
  - Migraine
  - Noncardiac chest pain
  - Pheochromocytoma
  - Recurrent abdominal pain
- Consider possible medication adverse effects: those from diet pills, antihistamines, albuterol, or caffeine.
- Consider avoidant/restrictive food intake disorder given this patient's anxiety around eating and fear of choking.

Keep in Mind: Diagnostic Changes Over Time

The clinician's diagnostic approach can be iterative. Readminister screening tools over time. Consider coexisting conditions if the patient is not responding as anticipated to evidence-based anxiety treatments. Although anxiety is not something children tend to "outgrow," they can go through intense, active periods and then feel better.

Because anxiety symptoms can wax and wane, the clinician will want to

- Readminister screening tools to compare current to prior scores; this a great way to monitor progress of symptoms or interference with functioning over time.
- Consider screening for comorbidities whenever symptoms affecting mental health are worsening or changing or a patient is not responding as expected for their diagnosis. This is a good time to use (or readminister) the PHQ-A to screen for depression and/or suicidal ideation.
  — If suicidal ideation is reported, consider using the ASQ and/or the C-SSRS to help identify risk, severity, and level of support needed for the patient.
- Consider a trauma screener such as the Child Trauma Screen (CTS) or the Child PTSD Symptom Scale for *DSM-5* (CPSS-5).

➤ **What tools could you use now to screen Sydney's new and worsening symptoms?**

You readminister the SCARED with Sydney, and you include the PHQ-A to assess her for depression and suicidal ideation (**Table 1-2**). The PHQ-A shows some mild depressive symptoms but no suicidal ideation. You determine that most of her symptoms are related to worsening anxiety, with symptoms of a panic disorder of moderate severity, and decide to move forward with a management plan. Her depressive symptoms will need ongoing monitoring, though.

Table 1-2. Sydney's Scores on the Readministered SCARED With the PHQ-A Included

Anxiety and Depression Subscales	Positive Score	Patient Score
SCARED		
Generalized Anxiety Disorder	9	13
Separation Anxiety Disorder	5	1
Social Anxiety Disorder	8	6
Panic Disorder/Significant Somatic Symptoms	7	24
Significant School Avoidance	3	6
Total Score	*>25*	*50*
PHQ-A		
Mild depression, no suicidal ideation endorsed	5	6

Abbreviations: PHQ-A, Patient Health Questionnaire-9 Modified for Adolescents; SCARED, Screen for Child Anxiety Related Emotional Disorders.

Management

Evidence-based treatment of anxiety includes cognitive behavioral therapy (CBT) and selective serotonin reuptake inhibitors (SSRIs).[8,9] The approach to anxiety treatment depends on the severity of symptoms. Severity is determined by the intensity of symptoms and degree of interference with functioning, as evidenced on screening tools and through clinical assessment.

- Mild anxiety: CBT
- Moderate anxiety: CBT + medication
- Severe anxiety: CBT + medication + consideration of referral for a higher level of care

Refer to Chapter 10, Anxiety and Anxiety Disorder, for the management of anxiety and the initiation of SSRIs.

A primary care clinician should be able to

- Facilitate brief interventions in the office.
- Initiate first-line medications as clinically indicated.
- Provide referrals to mental health specialists.
- Provide supportive monitoring until a mental health specialist is involved and the patient's condition is stable with medication.

➤ How often do you want to follow-up with Sydney?

This depends on the severity of her anxiety symptoms, whether she is taking medication, and whether she is also following up with a mental health specialist. Here is a general guideline for follow-up.

- Initial/acute phase (first 6 months): every 4 weeks
- Maintenance phase (6–12 months): every 3 months
- Discontinuation phase (12+ months): monitoring for several months during the tapering of medication

Consider scheduling nurse follow-up visits or telephone/virtual check-ins between visits.

Conclusion

Sydney's moderate anxiety responded well to a combined treatment approach of CBT and an SSRI. She continued to follow up with you in clinic every few months and you praised her hard work. She can routinely practice the brief interventions you taught her, and she challenged her anxious thoughts that were getting in the way of her success. She continued with therapy, receiving evidence-based treatment to target her anxiety symptoms and reduce her avoidance behavior. She now better understands her anxiety and the ways in which it affects her. She reports improvements in her sleep, mood, and appetite as well. On follow-up rating scales, you see marked improvement in her symptoms. Sydney's functioning has improved, and she can now dine out with friends without having somatic symptoms or panic attacks. When she does feel chest pain, she now has the tools she needs to help minimize the impact of her symptoms and does not avoid them.

Lessons Learned From Lightning

In the Lightning case (as somatic symptoms or panic disorder unfolds), patients can feel the physical manifestations of their psychological symptoms intensely throughout their body, so helping them understand the mind-body connection is an important part of their treatment. While physical disorders need to be ruled out, anxiety should always be included in the differential diagnosis for common childhood symptoms such as headaches, stomachaches, bed-wetting, and chest pain.

- Anxiety disorders are one of the most common and early presenting mental health concerns in children.[10]
- Comorbidities should be explored initially at diagnosis and iteratively if symptoms are not improving.
- The SCARED can help diagnose anxiety in children 8 years and older and will give the clinician subscale scores for some types of anxiety disorders, including panic disorder.
- Cognitive behavioral therapy is the first-line evidence-based treatment of mild to moderate anxiety.[8,9]
- Selective serotonin reuptake inhibitors are the first-line pharmacological treatment of moderate to severe anxiety.[6,7] Use a "start low, go slow" approach to initiation and screen the patient for suicidality.

Keywords: anxiety, chest pain, depression, panic disorder, somatic symptoms

Suggested Reading

Baum R, Campo J. Medically unexplained symptoms. In: Foy JM, ed. *Mental Health Care of Children and Adolescents: A Guide for Primary Care Clinicians*. American Academy of Pediatrics; 2018:649–659

Birmaher B, Brent DA, Chiappetta L, Bridge J, Monga S, Baugher M. Psychometric properties of the Screen for Child Anxiety Related Emotional Disorders (SCARED): a replication study. *J Am Acad Child Adolesc Psychiatry.* 1999;38(10):1230–1236 PMID: 10517055

Centre for Clinical Interventions. What is anxiety? Information sheet. Western Australian Department of Health. Accessed January 26, 2026. https://www.cci.health.wa.gov.au/~/media/CCI/Mental-Health-Professionals/Anxiety/Anxiety---Information-Sheets/Anxiety-Information-Sheet---01---What-is-Anxiety.pdf

Goodman R. The Strengths and Difficulties Questionnaire: a research note. *J Child Psychol Psychiatry.* 1997;38(5):581–586 PMID: 9255702

Kroenke K, Spitzer RL, Williams JBW. *Patient Health Questionnaire-9 (PHQ-9)*. APA PsycTests; 1999

Marroquin Y, Lewis J, Wallace W, et al. Outpatient behavioral health and primary care clinical pathway for the evaluation and treatment of anxiety disorder and obsessive-compulsive disorder. Children's Hospital of Philadelphia. Reviewed September 2021. Accessed January 26, 2026. https://www.chop.edu/clinical-pathway/anxiety-and-ocd-clinical-pathway

Murphy JM, Bergmann P, Chiang C, et al. The PSC-17: subscale scores, reliability, and factor structure in a new national sample. *Pediatrics.* 2016;138(3):e20160038 PMID: 27519444

Spitzer RL, Kroenke K, Williams JBW, Löwe B. A brief measure for assessing generalized anxiety disorder: the GAD-7. *Arch Intern Med.* 2006;166(10):1092–1097 PMID: 16717171

References

1. American Psychiatric Association. Generalized anxiety disorder. In: *Diagnostic and Statistical Manual of Mental Disorders*. 5th ed, text rev. American Psychiatric Association Publishing; 2022:250
2. American Psychiatric Association. Panic disorder. In: *Diagnostic and Statistical Manual of Mental Disorders*. 5th ed, text rev. American Psychiatric Association Publishing; 2022:253
3. American Psychiatric Association. Social anxiety disorder. In: *Diagnostic and Statistical Manual of Mental Disorders*. 5th ed, text rev. American Psychiatric Association Publishing; 2022:229
4. Duffee J, Szilagyi M, Forkey H, Kelly ET, Springer SH; American Academy of Pediatrics Council on Community Pediatrics; Council on Foster Care, Adoption, and Kinship Care; Council on Child Abuse and Neglect; and Committee on Psychosocial Aspects of Child and Family Health. Trauma-informed care in child health systems. *Pediatrics.* 2021;148(2):e2021052579 PMID: 34312294
5. Harris M, Fallot RD, eds. *Using Trauma Theory to Design Service Systems: New Directions for Mental Health Services*. Jossey-Bass; 2001
6. Yadav G, McNamara S, Gunturu S. Trauma-informed therapy. In: *StatPearls*. StatPearls Publishing; 2024. Updated August 16, 2024. Accessed January 26, 2026. https://www.ncbi.nlm.nih.gov/books/NBK604200

7. Chand SP, Marwaha R. Anxiety. In: *StatPearls*. StatPearls Publishing; 2023. Updated April 24, 2023. Accessed January 26, 2026. https://www.ncbi.nlm.nih.gov/books/NBK470361
8. Compton SN, Walkup JT, Albano AM, et al. Child/Adolescent Anxiety Multimodal Study (CAMS): rationale, design, and methods. *Child Adolesc Psychiatry Ment Health*. 2010;4:1 PMID: 20051130
9. Wehry AM, Beesdo-Baum K, Hennelly MM, Connolly SD, Strawn JR. Assessment and treatment of anxiety disorders in children and adolescents. *Curr Psychiatry Rep*. 2015;17(7):52 PMID: 25980507
10. Ramsawh HJ, Chavira DA, Stein MB. Burden of anxiety disorders in pediatric medical settings: prevalence, phenomenology, and a research agenda. *Arch Pediatr Adolesc Med*. 2010;164(10):965–972 PMID: 20921356

CHAPTER 2

Separation Anxiety

The Wave: Characterized by fluctuating symptoms that may vary by situation. Look out for waves that overwhelm the novice swimmers.

Presentation

Phoenix is a 14-year-old boy who lives in the city with his mother and grandmother. He has come to your office with his mother to discuss concerns about chronic fatigue. His mother notes that she has a hard time getting him out of bed in the morning and that it seems like he is moving in slow motion as he gets ready for school. His mother works as a home health aide overnight. She typically leaves for her shift around 8:00 pm and gets off work at 5:00 am. When she arrives home, she helps Phoenix get ready for school. Phoenix reports that after he is woken up, he has difficulty getting started and feels tired and sluggish. Because his mother works all night, she reports that she is on autopilot to get him out the door and will occasionally fall asleep before he leaves. Phoenix additionally reports that as he starts getting ready, he feels nauseous and sweaty and his heart starts racing. Sometimes he feels like he may faint but has never done so. He discloses feeling much better if he gets back into bed, especially knowing that his mother is home. However, he sometimes falls back asleep and misses school and his mother sometimes does not realize he has overslept until she wakes around lunchtime. While she enjoys eating lunch with him, she is worried about why he is so tired and about the implications on his grades, as she recently received a truancy letter for his unexcused absences. She remembers feeling very tired when she was his age and wonders if he has anemia, which she was diagnosed with as a young adult.

Review of Systems

- **Constitutional:** no fevers, weight loss/gain, or night sweats
- **HEENT:** no vision changes
- **Respiratory:** no cough or shortness of breath
- **Gastrointestinal:** no vomiting or diarrhea
- **Integumentary:** no rashes
- **Lymphatic:** no enlarged lymph nodes
- **Neurological:** no headaches

In addition, his growth, vital signs, and physical examination findings are entirely normal for his age.

Social History

- Strengths: kind, good friend
- School: average student, no support needed, but recently having trouble keeping up with work due to school absences
- Home: lives with mother and grandmother, no pets
- Activities: member of school soccer team in the fall
- Drugs: does not report using alcohol, tobacco products, or marijuana
- Emotions: often worries about things, has never been in therapy
- Sexuality: unsure about attraction, no sexual activity
- Safety: no guns in home, wears seatbelt, inconsistent sunscreen use, feels safe at home and in school

➤ **What do you think is causing Phoenix's fatigue, nausea, tachycardia, and diaphoresis?**

Differential Diagnosis

Phoenix's symptoms and family history raise concern for anemia, which his mom notes as her primary concern for the visit. However, he has no chronic disease associated with anemia, no reported blood loss, and no dietary restrictions noted that make anemia more likely.

- **Anemia:** Symptoms can include fatigue, malaise, and tachycardia, but he does not have any pallor, dizziness/lightheadedness, headache, or shortness of breath noted.
- **Vitamin deficiency:** A vitamin B_{12} deficiency can be associated with fatigue, nausea, and palpitations. There can also be associated neurological symptoms such as muscle weakness, numbness, balance issues, and paresthesia, but these are not reported.

Other diagnoses to consider include

- **Hypothyroidism:** Symptoms include fatigue, lethargy, and sluggishness. Phoenix does not have the symptoms of cold intolerance, hair loss, constipation, dry skin, high cholesterol level, bradycardia, or weight gain.
- **Epstein-Barr virus (EBV):** Symptoms often include fatigue, but they can also include fever, pharyngitis, enlarged lymph nodes, and rash, which Phoenix does not have. Adolescents are often symptomatic with EBV and may feel fatigued for weeks or months after the acute infection.
- **Pheochromocytoma:** Paroxysmal attacks of high blood pressure, tachycardia, sweating, and headaches, typically occurring in school-aged children and often genetic. While many of the symptoms come and go, high blood pressure is likely to be chronic.
- **Postural orthostatic tachycardia syndrome:** Often begins around puberty and is more common in girls than boys. Symptoms often include palpitations, chest discomfort, lightheadedness/dizziness/fainting, exercise intolerance, and extreme fatigue. The symptoms can be triggered by changing from a supine to standing position.
- **Lyme disease:** Early symptoms include a rash (erythema migrans) and flu-like symptoms (eg, headache, fatigue, swollen lymph nodes). Late-stage disease can include carditis, which causes palpitations.
- **Substance use disorder:** Cocaine use can cause dilated pupils, hyperactivity, tachycardia, diaphoresis, and nausea. Cannabis use can lead to nausea and tachycardia. Hallucinogens (eg, mushrooms, LSD, PCP) can cause symptoms of panic, including tachycardia, diaphoresis, and insomnia. Alcohol withdrawal is associated with weakness, diaphoresis, and tachycardia.
  - In addition to substances Phoenix could be using, consider medications or supplements he could be taking such as stimulants, decongestants (eg, pseudoephedrine), ginseng, isotretinoin, lidocaine, and diphenoxylate and atropine (ie, Lomotil).
- **Depression:** Poor sleep with daytime somnolence, acute change in school attendance, and psychomotor agitation or retardation can occur with depressive disorders. Remember that depression occurs in approximately 4% of children.[1]

- **Anxiety:** Tachycardia, nausea, fatigue, and diaphoresis can occur with anxiety disorders.
  - *Panic disorder:* Acute onset of tachycardia and sweating without an identified trigger could represent recurring panic attacks. To meet criteria for panic disorder, Phoenix would need to experience 1 or more attacks followed by at least 1 month of fear of another panic attack or significant maladaptive behaviors related to the attacks.
  - *Social anxiety disorder:* Is there excessive worry or distress about going to school or being in the presence of peers?
  - *Separation anxiety disorder:* Is there excessive worry or distress related to his mother's job and time away from home? Does he worry about her safety in a way that impedes his ability to sleep?
- **Trauma:** Past traumatic experiences can affect his feeling of safety and overall anxious presentation and sluggish demeanor.
- **Somatic symptom disorder:** There is a focus here on physical symptoms that is resulting in distress and interfering with daily functioning.

Keep in Mind: Coexisting Conditions

These diagnoses are not mutually exclusive; sometimes an organic etiology can exacerbate underlying anxiety or depression symptoms, or multiple diagnoses may be comorbid.

➤ **Is there any additional evaluation you would like to do to narrow down this differential diagnosis?**

Evaluation

- History: Assess for drug and/or alcohol use; ask additional family history questions about mental health, pheochromocytoma (multiple endocrine neoplasia, neurofibromatosis, and von Hippel-Lindau disease), autoimmune conditions (celiac disease and diabetes), diet (vitamin B_{12}, folate, and iron intake), and social stressors (bullying, family disturbances, trauma, environmental hazards, and exposure to violence).
  - ***Tip:*** *In the evaluation of symptoms that are reported as happening before school, it can be helpful to ask about the pattern of symptoms.*
    - *For example, ask the parent:* Do these symptoms happen in the mornings when there is no school (eg, holiday breaks, weekends, summer break)? Do the symptoms resolve as the day goes on, or do they recur later in the day? Do they happen every school day, or are there certain days of the week (ie, timed with a particular school activity or mode of transportation)? What was notable about the days when the symptoms did not occur?
    - *For example, ask the patient:* How do you feel when you go back to sleep and miss the day? Does it feel like relief? Do you wish things could be different?

- Vital signs: Blood pressure, heart rate, and orthostatic vital signs.
- Laboratory evaluation: Complete blood cell (CBC) count, ferritin level, thyrotropin (previously referred to as *thyroid-stimulating hormone*) with reflex to free thyroxine function, and EBV serology.
- Screening tools (refer to the Appendix for links to the tools online):
  — **Screen for Child Anxiety Related Emotional Disorders (SCARED):** A pediatric anxiety screener used for children 8 years and older. A total score of 25 or higher may indicate the presence of an anxiety disorder. Child and parent rating scale versions are available.
    - Additionally, this screener will give the clinician subscale scores, which may indicate a specific type of anxiety disorder such as generalized anxiety disorder, social anxiety disorder, panic, school anxiety, and separation anxiety.

  — **Generalized Anxiety Disorder-7 (GAD-7):** An efficient, 7-question self-report tool for youth aged 13 to 17 years for screening, diagnosis, and severity assessment of generalized anxiety disorder. The GAD-7 does not separate types of anxiety but provides a total score.
    - Cutoff scores are
      - 5–9—mild
      - 10–14—moderate
      - 15–21—severe
    - A score of 8 or higher is considered atypical and warrants further evaluation for the presence of an anxiety disorder.

The evaluation reveals that Phoenix is not using any medications or drugs, has normal blood pressure and orthostatic vital signs, and has unremarkable findings from laboratory evaluation, including CBC, ferritin level, thyroid function, and EBV serology. He completed the SCARED and scored a 30, which indicates the likelihood of the presence of an anxiety disorder. More specifically on the SCARED, he scored an 11 on the Separation Anxiety Disorder subscale and a 5 on the Significant School Avoidance subscale (Table 2–1). These are elevated subscale scores that are worth further exploration.

Table 2–1. Phoenix's Scores on the SCARED

Anxiety Subscales	Positive Score	Patient Score
Generalized Anxiety Disorder	9	10
Separation Anxiety Disorder	5	11
Social Anxiety Disorder	8	3
Panic Disorder/Significant Somatic Symptoms	7	1
Significant School Avoidance	3	5
Total Score	*≥25*	*>25*

Abbreviation: SCARED, Screen for Child Anxiety Related Emotional Disorders.

Keep in Mind: Screening Tools

Screening tools can be useful for identifying individuals who may be at increased risk for mental health concerns; however, they are not a substitute for a comprehensive diagnostic evaluation. Most screening tools are designed to be brief and sensitive to potential symptoms, which means they could fail to capture the full clinical context. As a result, findings from screening measures should be interpreted with caution and within the broader context of clinical judgment.

When a screening tool indicates a potential concern, it is important to follow up with a clinical interview to gather additional information regarding symptom presentation, duration, and functional impact. In many cases, a positive screening result should also prompt referral to an appropriate mental health specialist for a more comprehensive diagnostic assessment to determine whether diagnostic criteria are met and to guide appropriate treatment planning.

Additionally, if a patient scores high on a subscale, it can be helpful to review the specific question(s) within that subscale with the patient, by using specific prompts. In this case, the clinician should review the criteria for separation anxiety disorder and how it specifically affects Phoenix.

In the SCARED, the following questions are related to the Separation Anxiety Disorder subscale

4.	I get scared if I sleep away from home.
8.	I follow my mother or father wherever they go.
13.	I worry about sleeping alone.
16.	I have nightmares about something bad happening to my parents.
20.	I have nightmares about something bad happening to me.
25.	I am afraid to be alone in the house.
29.	I don't like to be away from my family.
31.	I worry that something bad might happen to my parents.

Once you review Phoenix's SCARED scores, you may try to elicit more history to support the diagnosis of separation anxiety disorder. According to the *Diagnostic and Statistical Manual of Mental Disorders, Fifth Edition, Text Revision* (*DSM-5-TR*), separation anxiety disorder involves excessive worry or fear when separation from a parent or caregiver happens.[2] If any of these items are strongly endorsed, the clinician can use the specific item as a point of discussion. For example, "I see you wrote that you worry about something bad happening to your parent. Can you tell me more about this?"

Back to the Case

You have an additional discussion with Phoenix and he reports feeling very nervous when his mother works overnight. She must travel to a different part of the city and take 2 buses to get there. Since she leaves before he is asleep, he has time to worry about her safety during her commute. He typically will call her when she gets there to check that she made it safely. If she forgets to call to check in, he will find things to do to stay awake until she calls. Although he is not alone at home, he finds that he has trouble "shutting off" his brain while he's trying to fall asleep, as he is worried something bad is going to happen to her on her commute. Eventually, he will fall asleep, but if he wakes up (eg, to use the bathroom), he will call her to check on her safety and will sometimes have difficulty going back to sleep. In the morning, once he knows she is on the way home, he will fall back asleep until his alarm wakes him up for school an hour or so later. He reports that he feels so much better saying this to you, as he has not talked about this worry, even with his mother. At the end of the visit, his mother asks if you can write a note allowing him to miss school to help avoid truancy.

Discussion

The clinical history, examination, laboratory findings, and scores on the SCARED screening tool suggest that Phoenix has a diagnosis of separation anxiety. While separation anxiety is developmentally appropriate up to around age 3 years, Phoenix's separation anxiety meets criteria in that it has caused functional impairment and significant distress and has lasted longer than 4 weeks.[2]

Management

Evidenced-based treatment of anxiety includes cognitive behavioral therapy (CBT) and selective serotonin reuptake inhibitors.[3,4] The approach to anxiety treatment depends on the severity of symptoms. For details on the treatment of anxiety, refer to Chapter 10, Anxiety and Anxiety Disorder.

A primary care clinician should be able to

- Facilitate brief interventions in the office, including using mental health screening tools.
- Initiate first-line medications as clinically indicated.
- Provide referrals to mental health specialists.
- Provide supportive monitoring until a mental health specialist is involved and the patient's condition is stable with medication.

●●● Communication Pearl ●●●
Emotion Validation

When a caregiver hears their child report concerns about their own safety, they are often quick to dismiss and reassure. For example,

- Child/teen: I don't like sleeping away from you because I'm afraid something might happen to you while I'm gone.
- Caregiver: Nothing is going to happen to me! I'm healthy and our house is safe!

While this reassurance is well-intentioned, the message it can send to children or teens is that their worry is invalid and, therefore, their feelings are invalid. Instead, suggest something such as the following example:

- Caregiver: I can only imagine how scary it is to worry I might not be here someday. I really appreciate you sharing this with me so I know this is bothering you. Let's think about some ways we can help you manage that worry when it arises.

This helps the child see that we empathize with their emotion and that we want to help share the burden in managing this uncomfortable feeling. As the adults in their life, we should be seen as safe places to discuss distressing feelings and sources of help when it is sought out.

When communicating with a child who feels anxious, it's helpful to remind a caregiver that denying the worry is like putting a bandage on a gaping wound. It will be beneficial to understand where the worry is coming from; to acknowledge that the fear can interfere with the child's important functioning, such as sleep; and to assure the child that together they will come up with a plan to address those feelings to help improve the child's functioning.

Brief interventions: You refer Phoenix for therapy with a mental health specialist and offer some brief interventions around sleep, school attendance, and relaxation that can help alleviate some of his anxiety.

- **Sleep hygiene**
  - Insomnia and nightmares can commonly occur with anxiety disorders. Phoenix should practice effective sleep hygiene, with a calming, screen-free bedtime routine; consistent bedtime; and 8 to 10 hours of sleep.
  - Since fear for his mother's safety is part of his stressors, perhaps help him and his mother create a point of communication either before bed or on waking, or at both, to help mitigate the worry and allow him to achieve better sleep.

- **Return to school**
  - — It is important that Phoenix face his fears and return to school every day. While therapy will help him feel emotionally ready to change his behavior, it is important to reframe to him the benefit of going to school as a way to face his fear. Additionally, returning to school will help him and his mom avoid additional punitive outcomes (eg, truancy).
  - — It will be in Phoenix's best interest if he does not receive a letter excusing his future absences to avoid truancy. While this will be a difficult conversation, excusing the absences will only prolong the cycle of avoidance that an anxiety disorder can cause.
- **Cognitive restructuring and relaxation**
  - — One technique that Phoenix will learn in therapy is something called *cognitive restructuring*, through which he will be able to change his unhelpful thoughts to more productive and helpful ones.[5] For example, when he wakes up to find that his mother has not returned from work, instead of thinking the worst-case scenario (eg, "Something bad has happened and I will never see her again"), he can change this thought to something that is the positive opposite (eg, "She is OK and I can text her now to check on her, as she is probably just on her way home").
  - — It can be helpful to teach Phoenix a quick way to relax when he is feeling tense and worried, such as box breathing. Have a way to describe this technique to him, such as "Breathe in slowly for 5 seconds through your nose and out slowly for 5 seconds from your mouth" or "smelling the flowers and blowing off the petals" and "blowing out the candles slowly" for younger children. Refer to Chapter 10, Anxiety and Anxiety Disorder, for further discussion.

••• Communication Pearl •••
Normalizing Anxious Thoughts

It's important to remember that everyone experiences anxiety or anxious thoughts from time to time. Anxiety is a natural fear response that helps keep us safe. Consider describing anxiety to a patient using the following example:

"Anxiety is like a wave in the ocean. Some days the ocean is calm and some days it is rough. On the calm days, you can manage it fine, but on the rough days, you need to know how to surf. The tools your therapist and I are teaching you are your surfboard. The waves are going to keep coming. I know you can swim, but I'm going to keep checking in until I know you can surf the big waves without me."

➤ How would this case be different if Phoenix were 3 years old?

It is developmentally appropriate for young children to have fears of separation from their caregiver or loved ones. These fears typically begin around 8 to 9 months of age and resolve by 3 years of age. Caregivers may first note that their infant looks fearful and cries when separated from them or does not want anyone but a specific caregiver to hold them. Separation fears in this age-group are inherently protective in nature, as children should want to be close to their caregiver. Between ages 2 and 3 years, toddlers start to understand that separation is normal and that their caregivers will eventually return. If a clinician is working with a family with a child exhibiting these types of fears, they can encourage the caregiver to use a phrase such as "Grown-ups come back" as a way to help the child understand what will happen.

It is also helpful for caregivers to communicate with their children ahead of separation about what is going to happen when they separate, what to expect during the time when they are apart, and what will happen when they reunite. For example, "Today, you will go to school, and although it will be hard to say goodbye, you are going to have a great day with your teachers and friends, and I will be right there to pick you up at the end of the day because grown-ups come back. Then we can play together when we get home." Additionally, if there are anticipated changes to normal separation, such as being picked up from school by a different person or having a babysitter, it is important to bring them up ahead of time so a child who feels anxious has time to process their emotions rather than experience the fear in real time.

After age 3 years, if the fear becomes excessive or extreme, it would be appropriate to look at separation anxiety disorder as part of a differential diagnosis. When thinking about separation anxiety disorder, clinicians can remember that the fears tend to go beyond a preference of caregiver proximity, becoming fears about safety, separation, and permanency of this separation.[6] Preschool and school-aged children may exhibit excessive clinginess and tantrums after the separation has occurred, plus significant dysregulation and difficulty calming down. As children mature, they can start to describe their own version of excessive worry or to display worried behavior such as clock/time checking or needing to frequently call/text caregivers when separated. They may also start to display anticipatory fears knowing that a separation is impending in the near future. They may decline leaving the house or engaging in social activities for fear of the safety of themselves or loved ones when separated.

Keep in Mind: Trauma-Informed Care and Culturally Sensitive Care

Using a trauma-informed care (TIC) approach, clinicians understand that a patient may have experienced traumatic events that have lasting effects on their health and wellness. In this case, Phoenix lives in an urban environment where exposure to violence may occur. Additionally, his mother's commute (eg, taking 2 buses across town after dark) may give Phoenix a valid reason to worry for her safety, although his level of concern may be excessive. Research has shown that parental shift work (eg, night shifts, rotating shifts) can have negative effects on youth mental health and behavior, including behavioral difficulties, adolescent depression, and decreased quality of the parent-child relationship.[7–9]

While Phoenix meets the criteria for a diagnosis, there will be many youth who have similar fears and worry about their parents' safety at the subclinical level, meaning their fears are distressing and interfering with daily functioning but have not reached a level of meeting criteria for a diagnosis. It is important to understand where fears are coming from and the effect it has on family functioning at any level.

The TIC approach pairs with providing culturally sensitive care as a way to address health disparities and promote health equity for children who may have experienced trauma.

Strategies for providing culturally sensitive care include[10,11]

- Understand and respect cultural backgrounds.
  - Listen for and use the family's own terms.
- Understand how the primary care clinician's helping role is perceived.
  - Connect families with trusted community resources.
- Provide linguistically competent care.
  - Do not use family members to provide interpretation.
  - Conduct visits in a family's preferred language.
- Provide care coordination for resources: transportation, finances, and interpreters.

➤ How often do you want to follow-up with Phoenix?

Once an anxiety disorder is diagnosed, regular follow-up is advised to monitor severity of symptoms, response to treatment, and ongoing screening for coexisting conditions. This depends on the severity of his anxiety symptoms, whether he is taking medication, and whether he is also following up with a mental health specialist. Here is a general guideline for follow-up.

- Initial/acute phase (first 6 months): every 4 weeks
- Maintenance phase (6–12 months): every 3 months
- Discontinuation phase (12+ months): monitoring for several months during the tapering of medication

➤ What tools could you use to screen his symptoms now and iteratively over time as he returns for follow-up visits?

- Readminister the SCARED. Following these scores over time can help assess severity of symptoms and monitor response to treatment.
- Remember that depression often co-occurs with anxiety, so you may also want to use the Patient Health Questionnaire-9 Modified for Adolescents (PHQ-A) to screen for depression and suicidality. Refer to the Appendix for the description of the PHQ-A and a link to the tool online.
- If trauma is suspected, consider a trauma screener such as the Child Trauma Screen (CTS) or the Child PTSD Symptom Scale for *DSM-5* (CPSS-5).
- Strengths and Difficulties Questionnaire (SDQ): A general behavioral screening questionnaire that focuses on emotional symptoms, conduct, hyperactivity/impulsivity, peer relationships, and prosocial behavioral concerns. Refer to the Appendix for the description of the SDQ and a link to the tool online.

Keep in Mind: Interference With Daily Functioning Check-In

For a quick measurement at each appointment, clinicians should ask patients to rate their level of interference with daily functioning and record the response in the patient's health record.

"On a scale of 1 to 10, 1 being that you are feeling your best, with almost no worry/sadness, and 10 being your worst, with worry/sadness that is too big to handle, where have you been most often in the past 2 weeks?"

Explain to caregivers that they can use this same scale to check in with their child, as it allows children to offer a measurement of their symptom severity without having to explain their feelings.

Conclusion

Phoenix has been meeting with a therapist and his separation anxiety has been responding well to CBT. He has participated in 6 sessions thus far. His mom followed the plan of gradually exposing him to school and other separations from her and now he attends school full-time and is able to fall asleep by 9:00 pm on nights his mother is working. On readministration of the SCARED rating scale, you see marked improvement in symptoms. Phoenix now has the tools he needs to manage his anxiety without medication; however, you discuss that they should follow up if symptoms ever recur or worsen.

Lessons Learned From the Wave

In the Wave case (as separation anxiety unfolds), the patient can be consumed by their anxiety, but the clinician can help them see that although the waves will keep coming, they have the tools they need to ride the waves, which will help them feel competent in managing their anxiety.

- Anxiety disorders are one of the most common and early presenting mental health concerns in children.[12]
- Separation anxiety is developmentally appropriate between ages 8 months and 3 years, but when it is excessive and persistent, it may reach the level of a diagnosable disorder and can occur at any age, including adolescence. Refer to the *DSM-5-TR* criteria when considering separation anxiety in a patient.[2]
- The SCARED can help diagnose anxiety in children aged 8 years and older and will give the clinician subscale scores for some types of anxiety disorders, including separation anxiety disorder. Screening questions can be used to lead into follow-up conversations (eg, "In the questionnaire, you circled that you really worry about your parents' safety when they are separated from you. Can you tell me more about that?").
- Cognitive behavioral therapy is the first-line evidence-based treatment of mild to moderate anxiety.[3]

Keywords: anxiety, cognitive restructuring, school avoidance, separation anxiety, truancy

Suggested Reading

Birmaher B, Brent DA, Chiappetta L, Bridge J, Monga S, Baugher M. Psychometric properties of the Screen for Child Anxiety Related Emotional Disorders (SCARED): a replication study. *J Am Acad Child Adolesc Psychiatry.* 1999;38(10):1230–1236 PMID: 10517055

Centre for Clinical Interventions. What is anxiety? Information sheet. Western Australian Department of Health. Accessed January 28, 2026. https://www.cci.health.wa.gov.au/~/media/CCI/Mental-Health-Professionals/Anxiety/Anxiety—Information-Sheets/Anxiety-Information-Sheet—01—What-is-Anxiety.pdf

Kroenke K, Spitzer RL, Williams JBW. *Patient Health Questionnaire-9 (PHQ-9).* APA PsycTests; 1999

Spitzer RL, Kroenke K, Williams JBW, Löwe B. A brief measure for assessing generalized anxiety disorder: the GAD-7. *Arch Intern Med.* 2006;166(10):1092–1097 PMID: 16717171

References

1. Bitsko RH, Claussen AH, Lichstein J, et al. Mental health surveillance among children—United States, 2013–2019. *MMWR Suppl.* 2022;71(2):1–42 PMID: 35202359
2. American Psychiatric Association. Separation anxiety disorder. In: *Diagnostic and Statistical Manual of Mental Disorders.* 5th ed, text rev. American Psychiatric Association Publishing; 2022:217
3. Compton SN, Walkup JT, Albano AM, et al. Child/Adolescent Anxiety Multimodal Study (CAMS): rationale, design, and methods. *Child Adolesc Psychiatry Ment Health.* 2010;4:1 PMID: 20051130
4. Wehry AM, Beesdo-Baum K, Hennelly MM, Connolly SD, Strawn JR. Assessment and treatment of anxiety disorders in children and adolescents. *Curr Psychiatry Rep.* 2015;17(7):52 PMID: 25980507
5. Stiede JT, Trent ES, Viana AG, Guzick AG, Storch EA, Hershfield J. Cognitive behavioral therapy for children and adolescents with anxiety disorders. *Child Adolesc Psychiatr Clin N Am.* 2023;32(3):543–558 PMID: 37201966
6. Kearney CA, Sims KE, Pursell CR, Tillotson CA. Separation anxiety disorder in young children: a longitudinal and family analysis. *J Clin Child Adolesc Psychol.* 2003;32(4):593–598 PMID: 14710468
7. Han WJ, Miller DP. Parental work schedules and adolescent depression. *Health Sociol Rev.* 2009;18(1):36–49 PMID: 20936086
8. Han WJ, Waldfogel J. Parental work schedules, family process, and early adolescents' risky behavior. *Child Youth Serv Rev.* 2007;29:1249–1266
9. Heymann J. *The Widening Gap: Why America's Working Families Are in Jeopardy and What Can Be Done About It.* Basic Books; 2000
10. Okoniewski W, Sundaram M, Chaves-Gnecco D, McAnany K, Cowden JD, Ragavan M. Culturally sensitive interventions in pediatric primary care settings: a systematic review. *Pediatrics.* 2022;149(2):e2021052162 PMID: 35098300
11. Health Care Toolbox. What is culturally-sensitive trauma-informed pediatric care? Accessed January 28, 2026. https://www.healthcaretoolbox.org/cultural-considerations#:~:text=Culturally%2DSensitive%20Trauma%2DInformed%20Care,beliefs%20about%20health%20and%20illness
12. Ramsawh HJ, Chavira DA, Stein MB. Burden of anxiety disorders in pediatric medical settings: prevalence, phenomenology, and a research agenda. *Arch Pediatr Adolesc Med.* 2010;164(10):965–972 PMID: 20921356

CHAPTER 3

Perfectionism

The Dandelion: Characterized by a delicate globe of seeds, fragile in the wind, falling apart or being blown away by ritualistic behaviors. Look out for an intensity in focus, negative self-talk, and inflexibility.

Presentation

Austin is an 8-year-old whose parents are bringing him to your office because they have concerns about rigidity of his behavior and its effect on his day-to-day functioning. Austin has always been a child who likes routines and orderliness. At home, he keeps his room tidy, and all his toys are organized in a special way that he likes. His parents have always felt proud that he takes pride in cleaning his room by making his bed and putting away his clean clothes, but small things can throw him off, such as toys being moved to a different spot or clothes being put into the wrong drawer. When this happens, he must correct the mistake before being able to move on with his day. Last week, they found Austin crying after dropping a block set that broke into pieces. They said he had a hard time forgiving himself and blew up at himself, calling himself stupid and wanting to throw away the blocks because he didn't deserve them. Afterward, he felt nauseous and refused to eat dinner because he was too upset.

At school, Austin is an exemplary student. For example, he follows rules, listens to teachers, and turns work in on time. Teachers have commented that he can often get stuck in checking his work, sometimes changing his answers to incorrect ones as he second-guesses himself. He tends to be the last child to finish a test during the allotted time, even though he has completed the work. He takes any missed points on tests as strong personal failures, believing that his teachers are going to be very angry at him and think he's stupid.

Outside of school, he plays baseball and shows dedication to his team by being the first person to show up to practice, always giving his all, and being the last to leave. In his most recent game, Austin missed a catch that lost the game for his team. Since then, he has wanted to skip practice because he either has a stomachache or has a headache. His parents are bringing him here to get him checked out, as this is happening multiple times per week and they are not sure whether there's something wrong or he is worried about letting down his team or seeming like a failure to them. Until recently, Austin's parents considered all these things personality quirks and thought they were qualities that benefited him. Now, Austin's parents are worried he might be autistic and wanted your input on next steps in evaluating him for autism.

Patient History and Review of Systems

- **Birth history:** full term, no complications
- **Medical history:** night terrors as a toddler
- **Family history:** paternal cousin on the autism spectrum
- **Social history:** lives at home with his mom, dad, and sister
- **Medications:** none
- **Constitutional:** no fevers, weight loss/gain, or night sweats
- **HEENT:** no vision or hearing concerns
- **Respiratory:** no cough or shortness of breath
- **Gastrointestinal:** no nausea/vomiting, diarrhea, constipation, or heartburn
- **Integumentary:** no rashes
- **Lymphatic:** no enlarged lymph nodes
- **Neurological:** no headaches, dizziness, or balance problems

➤ **Do you share the concern about autism spectrum disorder? What else might be contributing to his behaviors?**

Differential Diagnosis

Austin is demonstrating rigidity and inflexibility, perfectionism, self-criticism, somatic symptoms, and social dysfunction that are interfering with his functioning and causing distress.

- **Autism spectrum disorder[1]:** Characterized by social skills deficits, inflexible and logical thinking, restricted and repetitive behaviors (eg, focused interests, stimming such as hand flapping), and speech and communication deficits.
  - Austin does not demonstrate restricted, repetitive behaviors; developmental delays; or communication impairments. Not much is reported about his social interactions, so more information is needed about how he has developed socially, including engaging in social-emotional reciprocity, demonstrating nonspeaking/minimally speaking (previously referred to as *nonverbal*) communication, and developing and maintaining relationships. In the office, his eye contact, body language, ability to share joint attention and interest, and reciprocal social interactions can be observed.
- **Obsessive-compulsive disorder (OCD)[2]:** Characterized by obsessions and/or compulsions. Obsessions are recurring intrusive and inappropriate thoughts, impulses, or images that cause the child distress, and compulsions are the behavior that tries to counteract the obsessions.
  - In Austin's case, his need to clean his room could be a compulsion related to an obsession for cleanliness or order. Similarly, checking his work repeatedly could be a compulsion that counteracts his obsession with getting 100% on all assignments. However, compulsions with OCD are often connected to intrusive thoughts such as "Bad things that will happen" if the ritual or compulsion is not completed. Therefore, the person must complete the ritual rather than have a personal quirk or strong feeling of liking order or cleanliness.
- **Anxiety disorder:** Characterized by excessive fears or worries that can interfere with daily functioning.
  - Austin does seem to have many fears connected to performance and cleanliness/orderliness. Further evaluation for a specific anxiety disorder could be warranted.

Keep in Mind: Obsessive-Compulsive Disorder and Anxiety Disorder

In the *Diagnostic and Statistical Manual of Mental Disorders, Fifth Edition, Text Revision* (*DSM-5-TR*), the most recent revision, OCD was removed as a category within the anxiety disorder category and given its own class called "Obsessive-Compulsive and Related Disorders." Therefore, an individual could meet criteria for OCD alone, anxiety disorder alone, or OCD and anxiety disorder together. Additionally, given that the 2 disorders used to be under the same class, their symptoms can overlap and are often comorbid.

- **Pediatric acute-onset neuropsychiatric syndrome (PANS):** The acute onset of neuropsychiatric symptoms (PANS) is unknown but is theorized to be triggered by recent infections or autoimmune conditions. This umbrella term includes pediatric autoimmune neuropsychiatric disorders associated with streptococcal infections (PANDAS).
  - The symptoms of PANS include the unusually abrupt and dramatic onset of OCD or restrictive food intake with a concurrent and abrupt onset of severe neuropsychiatric symptoms from at least 2 of 7 categories, including anxiety; emotional lability and/or depression; irritability, aggression, and/or severe oppositional behaviors; developmental regression; deterioration in school performance; sensory or motor abnormalities including heightened sensitivity to sensory stimuli, hallucinations, dysgraphia, and complex motor and/or vocal tics; and somatic signs and symptoms, including sleep disturbances, enuresis, and urinary frequency, that are not better explained by a known neurological or medical disorder.[3] PANS is not in the *DSM-5-TR* and remains a diagnosis of exclusion.
- **Attention-deficit/hyperactivity disorder (ADHD):** Children struggle with attention and focus, with some showing mainly only deficits in attention skills (ADHD—predominately inattentive presentation), some showing significant hyperactivity and impulsivity (ADHD—predominately hyperactive/impulsive presentation), or some showing both (ADHD—combined).
  - Children with ADHD can exhibit repetitive behaviors, sometimes associated with their hyperactivity. Also, while individuals with ADHD are inattentive with some activities, they can be preoccupied with preferred, enjoyable activities, which caregivers sometimes describe as "hyperfocused." The inattention of ADHD is different from the worry or rumination of anxiety that results in inattention.
    - In Austin's case, there are no reports of hyperactivity. He may demonstrate some hyperfocus on cleanliness and organization but does not seem to demonstrate inattention elsewhere. He has no reported issues with attention at school, but children with ADHD need to have symptoms in at least 2 settings, which typically include home and school.
- **Twice exceptional[4]:** Children are highly gifted in some areas while having learning difficulties in other areas. For example, they may be gifted in math and have inattention associated with ADHD or may be gifted in musical ability and have dyslexia. Often the strengths of these children can make it harder to uncover their struggles, and learning disabilities can go undiagnosed. Alternatively, a child's self-esteem and confidence can be diminished by their learning disability, leading to their giftedness going unrecognized and unencouraged.

— In this case, Austin shows high achievement in academics and demonstrates intensity of focus on preferred activities, which are typical of gifted children, but he also struggles with social skills, which may be a sign of a neurodevelopmental condition such as autism or ADHD.

➤ **Based on the conversation so far with Austin and his parents, what are some of the questions you could ask to tease out the diagnosis of autism versus anxiety versus OCD?**

Evaluation

Q: Austin, does your need to clean your room get in your way of doing other things that you want to do? Have you ever felt like something really bad would happen if you left your room messy or if things were out of order?

A: No, I like having a tidy room and I hate when my parents put things in the wrong drawers. If I wasn't cleaning my room, I would probably be organizing my backpack.

- The symptoms of OCD are ego-dystonic, whereas the symptoms of autism are ego-syntonic. That means that in people with OCD, the symptoms are incongruous with their self-image, whereas in those with anxiety and autism, the symptoms are in sync with their sense of self. So, in Austin's case, his symptoms are in line with his sense of self, making diagnoses such as anxiety and autism more likely than OCD, in which he would feel compelled to complete these tasks or else something bad might happen.

Q: Mom or Dad, was Austin's development delayed?

A: No, Austin met all his early developmental milestones on or before schedule according to the DSM-5-TR. *His speech was always sophisticated for his age. In fact, this year he is going to be tested for the gifted program at school.*

- Inconsistency in development can be a major clue to the diagnosis of autism. Individuals on the autism spectrum may have had regressions, delays, or large variations in development. Social and communication delays are part of the *DSM-5-TR* criteria.[1] If still needing to seek further clarification, the clinician can ask about Austin's social skills and whether he has difficulty making or maintaining friendships.

Q: Mom or Dad, how is Austin with other kids? Does he make friends easily or maintain friendships?

A: Austin has never really put a lot of effort into making friends, but other kids seem to like him. He had playdates when he was younger, and they always seemed to play well together. He has 1 to 2 close friends, but he feels like he has too much homework or sports practice to really hang out with others. He's also never slept over at someone's house.

- Another major component of autism spectrum disorder is deficits in social skills. It sounds as if Austin's social relationships are not a priority for him, but they are not a deficit either.

Q: Austin, what is making baseball hard for you?

A: I like things to happen in a certain order. I need to put on my batting glove and touch the Velcro band 3 times. Then I twist my bat and tap my shoe 3 times. But sometimes the umpire gets in my way and then I have to start over, but my coach doesn't let me and I get upset. And the other kids make fun of me if I get upset and that makes me mad.

- A preoccupation with order is a characteristic of OCD. In this case, the thoughts of what Austin needs to do are his obsessions and the acts of touching the band and tapping his bat are his compulsions. Although Austin's parents were reading his frustration as being about letting his team down at bat, it was actually about not being able to complete his rituals. These behaviors could be rituals and compulsions that are a diagnostic clue for OCD, but given they are occurring only in the context of sports, they could be a sport-related ritual. A big distinction will be whether this ritual causes distress, interferes with functioning, and is driven by fear of negative outcomes if not performed.

➤ What screening tools could you use to help you in your diagnostic approach?

- Autism
  - **Modified Checklist for Autism in Toddlers (M-CHAT):** A validated brief parent-report screening tool for children aged 16 months to 30 months who may be at risk for autism spectrum disorder. If there is clinician concern after scoring, the child should be referred to a specialist for full diagnostic evaluation.
- Anxiety
  - **Screen for Child Anxiety Related Emotional Disorders (SCARED):** A pediatric anxiety screener used for children 8 years and older. A total score of 25 or higher may indicate the presence of an anxiety disorder. Child and parent rating scale versions are available.
    - Additionally, this screener will give the clinician subscale scores, which may indicate a specific type of anxiety disorder such as generalized anxiety disorder, social anxiety disorder, panic, school anxiety, and separation anxiety.

Keep in Mind: Screening Tools Versus Diagnostic Assessments

As mentioned in Chapter 2, Separation Anxiety, there is a difference between a screening tool and a diagnostic assessment. A screening tool is brief, and it can be used initially, as well as iteratively, to monitor symptoms. It does not replace the need for an assessment, which is a comprehensive diagnostic process that helps guide diagnosis, severity, and treatment planning.

For example, in this case, you can use the M-CHAT to assess for symptoms connected to autism spectrum disorder. If the disorder is indicated, then it is imperative to have your patient follow up with a diagnostic assessment with a trained professional who may give a gold standard assessment tool such as the Autism Diagnostic Observation Schedule (ADOS) or Autism Diagnostic Interview, Revised (ADI-R).

- Obsessive-compulsive disorder
  - **Children's Yale-Brown Obsessive-Compulsive Scale (CY-BOCS):** A clinician-administered, semi-structured interview used to assess for the presence and severity of obsessive-compulsive symptoms in children and adolescents aged 6 to 17 years. It generates separate and total severity scores.
  - **Children's Obsessional Compulsive Inventory-Revised-Self Report (ChOCI-R-S):** A self-report questionnaire to assess the presence and severity of obsessive-compulsive symptoms in children and adolescents aged 7 to 17 years, including washing, checking, ordering, obsession, hoarding, and neutralizing.

Refer to the Appendix for links to the tools online.

➤ Is perfectionism a disorder?

Perfectionism as a personality trait can lead individuals to excel and reach goals successfully.[5] These individuals tend to have routines that they rigidly follow, but this behavior does not cause them distress. They also have high expectations of themselves and others, but this thinking may drive them toward success. Those with perfectionist tendencies like to be in control but can recover when they lose control or do not meet high expectations.

There is no official diagnosis of perfectionism. However, perfectionism can be a strong contributor to anxiety and depressive disorders in childhood, as the pressure to succeed can potentially place children at risk for failure and interference with functioning. It can also be a precursor to OCD, which can be diagnosed later in life.[6] Perfectionism as a manifestation of an anxiety disorder occurs when the perfectionism interferes with functioning (eg, relationships are affected, sleep is disrupted, and tasks are avoided for fear of failure) and the perfectionism is causing distress (eg, negative self-talk, low self-esteem).

In these cases, the clinician would want to proceed with treating it as an anxiety disorder (refer to Chapter 10, Anxiety and Anxiety Disorder). Some research indicates that perfectionism may be a predictor of OCD.[6,7] Therefore, while perfectionistic tendencies can be helpful for certain individuals, it is important to assess for prevalence, impact, and interference to better understand the difference between performance-enhancing and problematic perfectionism.

••• Communication Pearl •••
Strengths-Based Communication

A patient with perfectionistic tendencies likely holds themselves to high standards and is worried about disappointing you, especially if you have had a longitudinal relationship. In clinic, this may be a child who gives you the "right" answer to every question or who, every time you share data (eg, vital signs, growth charts), nervously asks, "Is that good?!" As they become adolescents, this perfectionism may limit their openness to share mistakes or to disclose health-related behaviors that they think would disappoint you, such as substance use or sexual behaviors. Therefore, it's important to use language that is nonjudgmental, open-ended, and strengths based.

Following the lessons of Kenneth Ginsburg, MD, MSEd, we should praise the communication and relationship in addition to the content, such as "Thank you for sharing that with me" in addition to "I'm so proud of your focus on school work," so they will be as willing to share the good as the bad.[8] Using a strengths-based approach, you can focus on what the patient tells you they are doing well and help coach them to see how their health-risk behaviors may harm them. For example, Dr Ginsburg suggests, "Let's talk about what might be getting in the way of being your best self."[8] Pediatric clinicians can model these communication skills for caregivers, as well as share a useful resource (https://parentandteen.com).

Back to the Case

Sometimes there is no diagnosis.

We have learned that Austin's symptoms are ego-syntonic, his early developmental history was normal, and he has a preoccupation with order. You suspect that anxiety might be playing a role in Austin's diagnostic picture, so you choose to have him complete the SCARED. His total score is a 22, which does not meet criteria for the presence of an anxiety disorder. However, when you take a closer look at the items he answered as true for him, they fall into the categories of fear of making mistakes, performance-related fears both in school and with peers, and worries about not meeting standards or disappointing others. He gets frustrated easily and has meltdowns. He also has difficulty completing his tasks if he cannot

Back to the Case (*continued*)

complete his rituals or maintain the type of orderliness that he feels compelled to keep. All of this taken together, Austin does not meet criteria for an anxiety disorder, OCD, ADHD, or autism, yet the constellation of symptoms continues to interfere with daily functioning at home and at school. This case describes a set of symptoms known as perfectionism, with some subthreshold anxiety, which is typically seen as a factor in other disorders but not often seen as a diagnosis itself.

Keep in Mind: Not All Patient Encounters Have to End With a Diagnosis to Be Successful

There may not be a diagnosis in the *DSM-5-TR* for every patient. However, clinicians and families can discuss symptoms, management, psychoeducation, brief interventions in the office setting, compassionate communication, and referrals for appropriate evidence-based treatment. It is also important to discuss risk factors for the development of mental health disorders and equally important to highlight protective factors that may mitigate worsening symptoms.

In cases such as this, it can seem frustrating if there is no official diagnosis, yet symptoms are interfering enough to cause concern. It is important to discuss your differential diagnosis with Austin and his family so they can not only understand how perfectionism is interfering with his functioning but also maintain vigilance for other disorders, such as anxiety and OCD, that could become more predominant diagnoses later in life.

➤ **Should Austin's parents pursue a diagnostic evaluation for autism?**

Discussion

Given the history provided, it is unlikely that Austin is autistic; therefore, a diagnostic evaluation is probably unnecessary. However, some of his perfectionistic tendencies seem to interfere with his social skills, as he is too consumed with worry about making mistakes to work on maintaining his friendships. This, along with the rigidity and orderliness, can seem like mannerisms similar to those of a child with mild autism. He may benefit from working with an occupational therapist in addition to a mental health specialist.

It is important to think through how to communicate this rationale to the parents. It is paramount to make sure the parents feel that their concerns were heard and validated. When providing this feedback, it can be helpful to say something like "I noticed you were concerned that Austin may have autism. Before I talk more about this, I'd like to understand why you mentioned autism and what you understand about autism." This will likely begin a conversation to understand how the parents view Austin's symptoms and how to align your understanding of the clinical presentation of diagnostic symptoms for autism, while allowing the parents to feel that you appreciated their concerns.

➤ What are some common coexisting conditions with OCD?

Among children and adolescents, OCD commonly co-occurs with other anxiety disorders, learning disorders, and disruptive behavior disorders.[2] In fact, coexisting conditions are common, including ADHD, Tourette syndrome, trichotillomania, body dysmorphia, and habits such as nail biting.[2,8–10]

Management

Even though there is no formal diagnosis in this case, there is still an ongoing need for management of his symptoms. A primary care clinician should be able to

- Facilitate brief interventions in the office setting and provide interval rating scales to monitor for changes in symptoms and interference with daily functioning.
- Initiate first-line medications as clinically indicated.
- Provide referrals to mental health specialists.
- Provide supportive monitoring until a mental health specialist is involved and the patient's condition is stable with medication.

Austin's parents want to know whether they should encourage him to attend baseball practices even though they cause him some distress.

Yes, children with perfectionistic tendencies sometimes avoid situations in which they may make mistakes. Taking risks and making mistakes are part of human development and crucial components of learning. For dealing with stressful situations and the internal chaos that fear of making mistakes can cause, it is important to help Austin learn relaxation and coping skills. Some age-appropriate ways to describe relaxation techniques include imagining a balloon inside the belly: "When you breathe in (inhale), the balloon gets bigger, and when you breathe out (exhale), it gets smaller." Pair this with a calming count such as "Breathe in for the count of 5 and make that balloon get really big and now breathe out for the count of 5 and feel it get smaller." Austin can also be encouraged to have a calming phrase that he can repeat to himself when he is trying to relax, such as "Mistakes are a part of life; I will be OK and I can learn from this."

It is important to encourage the family to continue with Austin's sports commitment. One of the greatest contributors to anxiety is called the *cycle of avoidance*. When Austin leaves baseball practice, his stomachache and headache likely go away. In time, he learns to avoid doing the things that cause those stomachaches and headaches (ie, the things that seem scary or make him feel sick). However, that cycle can negatively contribute to his sense of self, as he does not learn that he is able to do these things, even if they are hard or if he makes mistakes. It is important for Austin to develop a sense of control over his fears and perfectionistic traits, and that is best achieved by working through difficult things, not avoiding them.

Austin's parents describe his sister as a perfectionist too. Knowing this family has another child with perfectionism, the clinician may want to discuss with them the importance they place on grades and how they message this to their children. Many parents equate grades with success, and children tie this to their self-worth and value. As school becomes more challenging, stress and anxiety increase to reach escalating achievement goals and avoid failures and disappointments. The clinician can explain to parents that allowing children to realize that everyone makes mistakes is an important lesson and can help their child build resilience that will serve them better in the long term.

Brief interventions: For children with high achievement or those with perfectionistic tendencies, clinicians can discuss the importance of a growth mindset, which is the belief that our abilities are not fixed and can be improved through effort and learning. For their parents, some tips include[11]

- **Praise the effort and process, not the grades.**
  - This could include "You worked so hard on that project" or "I know how much you studied for that test." This focuses on the process of learning and growing, which they can apply to their next challenge, rather than the grade, which is already in the past and offers little feedback.
- **Build autonomy.**
  - Parents must let adolescents learn to manage their own tasks and make their own decisions. As hard as it can be as a parent to sit back and watch when you think you know the answer, this autonomy helps them develop confidence and self-esteem in their work.
- **Model healthy behaviors.**
  - As clinicians, we often encourage parents to share their own mistakes and how they recovered from them. Adults aren't perfect and we should show the children in our lives how we learn and grow from our setbacks as well!

Conclusion

As previously discussed, perfectionism and anxiety are linked. Therefore, helping Austin and his family better understand anxiety, its effect on functioning, and the course of treatment will help them monitor his psychosocial functioning as he continues to mature. You may want to do active monitoring for Austin, which includes checking in every few months. In the meantime, provide psychoeducation on healthy habits to promote positive well-being, including exercise, healthy eating, sleep hygiene, relaxing activities, goal setting, gratitude practices, and staying connected. You should also make sure he knows about the 988 Lifeline for mental health emergencies.

Lessons Learned From the Dandelion

In the Dandelion case (as perfectionism unfolds), the patient may seem perfect, or as if they are working at perfecting something, but if their perfectionism is causing distress or interfering with functioning, the clinician should consider the possibility that this behavior is driven by anxiety, OCD, or other mental health disorders. While perfectionism can lead to individuals excelling, it may also contribute to anxiety and depression developing. Many individuals that are high functioning are praised for their perfectionistic habits and, over time, feel the need to meet increasingly higher standards, which can create anxiety and lead to distress and interference with functioning. Not meeting those high standards can lead to feelings of sadness and worthlessness. While some perfectionism can appear rigid and inflexible, it is important to ascertain whether these symptoms are aligned with an individual's sense of self or causing fear, as in the case of compulsions in individuals with OCD.

- Screen individuals with perfectionism for anxiety and depression.
- In the *DSM-5-TR*, OCD is no longer a subset of anxiety disorder and is its own diagnosis, but these diagnoses have many similarities and are often coexisting.[2]
- The symptoms of OCD are ego-dystonic, whereas the symptoms of anxiety are ego-syntonic.
- Coexisting conditions are common with OCD and include anxiety, ADHD, Tourette syndrome, learning disorders, and body dysmorphia.[2,9,10]
- Using strengths-based communication may help adolescent patients be open to communicating their challenges as well as acknowledging their successes, as all people need to hear things that are going well or ways in which one can see effort.[8]

Keywords: anxiety, autism, OCD, PANS, perfectionism, strengths-based communication

Suggested Reading

Affrunti NW, Woodruff-Borden J. Perfectionism in pediatric anxiety and depressive disorders. *Clin Child Fam Psychol Rev.* 2014;17(3):299–317 PMID: 24481881

Hirota T, King BH. Autism spectrum disorder: a review. *JAMA.* 2023;329(2):157–168 PMID: 36625807

Pozza A, Albert U, Dèttore D. Perfectionism and intolerance of uncertainty are predictors of OCD symptoms in children and early adolescents: a prospective, cohort, one-year, follow-up study. *Clin Neuropsychiatry.* 2019;16(1):53–61 PMID: 34908939

Shatkin JP. *Child and Adolescent Health: A Practical All-in-One Guide.* WW Norton & Co; 2015

Ye HJ, Rice KG, Storch EA. Perfectionism and peer relations among children with obsessive-compulsive disorder. *Child Psychiatry Hum Dev.* 2008;39(4):415–426 PMID: 18338246

References

1. American Psychiatric Association. Autism spectrum disorder. In: *Diagnostic and Statistical Manual of Mental Disorders.* 5th ed, text rev. American Psychiatric Association Publishing; 2022:56–57
2. American Psychiatric Association. Obsessive-compulsive disorder. In: *Diagnostic and Statistical Manual of Mental Disorders.* 5th ed, text rev. American Psychiatric Association Publishing; 2022:266
3. Board of Directors. Pediatric acute-onset neuropsychiatric syndrome (PANS): clinical report. *Pediatrics.* 2025;155(3):e2024070334 PMID: 39676248
4. Arky B. Twice-exceptional kids: both gifted and challenged. Child Mind Institute. December 18, 2025. Accessed March 23, 2026. https://childmind.org/article/twice-exceptional-kids-both-gifted-and-challenged
5. Stoeber J, Rambow A. Perfectionism in adolescent school students: relations with motivation, achievement, and well-being. *Pers Individ Dif.* 2007;42(7):1379–1389
6. Lunn J, Greene D, Callaghan T, Egan SJ. Associations between perfectionism and symptoms of anxiety, obsessive-compulsive disorder and depression in young people: a meta-analysis. *Cogn Behav Ther.* 2023;52(5):460–487 PMID: 37194469
7. Shafran R, Mansell W. Perfectionism and psychopathology: a review of research and treatment. *Clin Psychol Rev.* 2001;21(6):879–906 PMID: 11497211
8. Ginsburg KR, Kinsman SB, eds. *Reaching Teens: Strength-Based Communication Strategies to Build Resilience and Support Healthy Adolescent Development.* American Academy of Pediatrics; 2014
9. Masi G, Millepiedi S, Mucci M, Bertini N, Pfanner C, Arcangeli F. Comorbidity of obsessive-compulsive disorder and attention-deficit/hyperactivity disorder in referred children and adolescents. *Compr Psychiatry.* 2006;47(1):42–47 PMID: 16324901
10. Walitza S, Melfsen S, Jans T, Zellmann H, Wewetzer C, Warnke A. Obsessive-compulsive disorder in children and adolescents. *Dtsch Arztebl Int.* 2011;108(11):173–179 PMID: 21475565
11. Lahey J. *The Gift of Failure: How the Best Parents Learn to Let Go So Their Children Can Succeed.* HarperCollins; 2016

CHAPTER 4

Substance Use

The Leaf: Characterized by a change in behavior. Look out for a strong influence of peers, social norms, and culture, as well as behavioral signs of shame and stigma.

Presentation

Madison is a 17-year-old who has been your patient since birth, and you also know her in your personal community outside the clinic. As a part of her adolescent health supervision visit, you use the SSHADESS framework to guide your clinical assessment.[1] Madison appears to be a reliable self-reporter and provides the following social history:

- **S**trengths: Likes music and singing; considers herself a good sister and friend.
- **S**chool: Grades have started to decline recently: was an A/B student, now has Cs in multiple classes, but thinks she can bring those up.
- **H**ome: She currently lives with her mom and 19-year-old brother. Her parents previously had an emotionally abusive relationship, before they divorced when she was 7 years old. Her dad is inconsistently in her life now. Her older brother is off at college and comes home on breaks.
- **A**ctivities: Her family is involved in their local church, and she sings in the choir; she also hangs out with friends after school and plays basketball recreationally.
- **D**rugs: She responds that she does not use alcohol, tobacco products, or drugs other than cannabis. She vapes once a month at school in the bathroom with friends. They usually do this when there's a pep rally at school, or they may vape at a party on the weekend. She does not feel like her use is out of control or interfering with necessary obligations or school.

- **E**motions: Her mom describes her as having been shy her whole life. When she was 7, her mother was concerned about the divorce and enrolled her in therapy, which she did for a year. She shares no history of anxiety or depression. She reports stressors in her life that are related to her school performance. No trouble sleeping. Normal appetite.
- **S**exuality: Attracted to men; no sexual activity.
- **S**afety: Feels safe at home and school; no bullying; no guns in her home; no suicidal or homicidal ideation; has not been in any fights; no history of physical or sexual abuse.

After reviewing her SSHADESS history, you are concerned about her monthly cannabis use and declining grades in school.

➤ **What is in your differential diagnosis?**

Differential Diagnosis

- **Substance use disorder (SUD)**
- **Learning disability**
- **Anxiety**
- **Depression**

It is important to identify reasons why Madison might be using marijuana. Common reasons youth use psychoactive substances include

- To fit in
- Peer pressure
- Expectations that use will be pleasurable
- As a form of risk-taking or stimulation seeking
- To relax
- To relieve anxiety
- To improve mood
- To relieve symptoms of a mental health disorder

In general, regardless of the substance being used, the clinician will want to ask about

- Age at initiation
- Frequency of use and last time used
- Typical amount consumed

- Problems associated with use, including impact on home, school, or social life
- Quit attempts and, if so, associated withdrawal symptoms
- Motivation to quit or change substance use behavior
- Riding/driving under the influence

Evaluation

In addition to the SSHADESS framework, there are other screening instruments that clinicians can use to assess a patient for substance use, including

- **Screening to Brief Intervention (S2BI):** A 7-item evidence-based, brief screening tool used to identify substance use risk among adolescents aged 12 to 17.
- **Brief Screener for Tobacco, Alcohol, and other Drugs (BSTAD):** A brief screening tool used to identify substance use risk among adolescents aged 12 to 17; the questionnaire assesses the number of days in the past year where substances were used, including tobacco/nicotine, alcohol, marijuana, and other drugs.
- **National Institute on Alcohol Abuse and Alcoholism (NIAAA) Alcohol Screening and Brief Intervention for Youth:** A 2-item validated, brief screening tool for youth aged 9 to 18 that assesses alcohol use and peer drinking behaviors in the past year; the scale is used to identify risk for alcohol-related problems and guidance for intervention.
- **CRAFFT (Car, Relax, Alone, Forget, Family/Friends, Trouble):** A screening and assessment tool for adolescents and young adults aged 12 to 21 for alcohol- and drug-related risk behaviors. This tool has a 9-item questionnaire and interview section.
- **Alcohol Use Disorders Identification Test (AUDIT):** A 10-item screening tool that assesses for risk of substance use issues including alcohol consumption, drinking behaviors, and alcohol-related problems for adolescents and adults.

Whichever method is used, clinicians should screen for problems associated with substance use and its effect on the patient's daily functioning at home, in school, and with peers. Questions should focus on age at initiation, frequency of use, and typical amount consumed.

Many clinicians have begun providing universal screening for depression, anxiety, and suicidal ideation at all adolescent visits. If these are not already incorporated into the patient evaluation, consider adding screenings for depression (Patient Health Questionnaire-9 Modified for Adolescents [PHQ-A]), anxiety (Screen for Child Anxiety Related Emotional Disorders [SCARED] or Generalized Anxiety Disorder-7 [GAD-7]), or suicidal ideation (the Ask Suicide-Screening Questions [ASQ] or Columbia-Suicide Severity

Rating Scale [C-SSRS]) whenever seeing a patient with substance use, as these are common coexisting conditions. Refer to the Appendix for brief descriptions of the tools and links to them online.

Keep in Mind: Confidentiality With Teens

It is important to review confidentiality with adolescent patients. While clinicians often meet with the adolescent alone for a confidential visit, it is important to discuss the limits of confidentiality, including that any concerns about safety will be shared with the caregiver, in particular if anyone is hurting them, there is self-injury or suicidal ideation, or they are hurting anyone else. Stating this at the beginning helps set expectations about what can be shared with caregivers (ie, abuse, suicidal ideation, homicidal ideation) and what cannot be shared. Clinicians should explain that they and the patient's caregivers have a shared goal of keeping them safe.

In this case, even though the patient and her family have been known to the clinician for many years, the clinician should stress that the patient's information remains private. However, when managing substance use, engaging families can be an important part of the treatment. It may be helpful for the clinician in this case to partner with Madison to see if she would be open to including her mother in this discussion. She may want to talk with her mom about this but be afraid to do so or not know how to start. Clinicians can serve as a bridge for patients and their caregivers to have this conversation in a safe and healthy way.

Back to the Case: Substance Use

You use the S2BI because it has an easy-to-use website and identifies the likelihood of an SUD using *Diagnostic and Statistical Manual of Mental Disorders, Fifth Edition, Text Revision* (*DSM-5-TR*) criteria.[2] You learn that in the past year, Madison typically uses her marijuana vape monthly in the bathroom at school or on the weekend at a party. This puts her in the "higher-risk" category, based on frequency of use. We also know she has evidence of declined functioning based on her academic performance.

The *DSM-5-TR* does include individual diagnoses for different types of SUDs, including cannabis use disorder. The criteria for cannabis use disorder include a problematic pattern of cannabis use leading to clinically significant impairment or distress, as manifested by at least 2 of the 11 diagnostic criteria (eg, a persistent desire or unsuccessful efforts to control cannabis use, and recurrent cannabis use results in failure to fulfill major obligations at work, home, or school) occurring within a 12-month period.[3] Refer to the *DSM-5-TR* for the full criteria.

Back to the Case (*continued*)

After using your assessment tools and discussing the past year with Madison, you note she does not meet *DSM-5-TR* criteria for cannabis use disorder, but she does have problematic use in that she meets at least 1 of the criteria. The other criteria are hard to assess at this time. When you express this to Madison, she says she doesn't know why you are asking so many questions about her vaping because everyone does it and marijuana isn't a big deal. Madison brings up a common issue of how societal views of marijuana and vape use have changed, including visibility and legality. This brings up an excellent question regarding the meaning and impact of daily or regular use.

➤ **How common is cannabis use among adolescents and how prevalent is cannabis use disorder? What does addiction mean among teenagers?**

Discussion: Substance Use

According to the *DSM-5-TR*, the prevalence of cannabis use disorder among youth aged 12 to 17 years is 2.7% to 3.1% and the onset of cannabis use disorder is highest in adolescence.[3] Although in most youth who use cannabis, a disorder will not develop, use is not without risk. Those who use cannabis 1 to 2 times per month are more likely to have negative impacts on academic performance, emotional state, and emotional regulation.[4] Perceived risk of marijuana use by youth is low, likely because of legalization and decriminalization over the years, as well as representation in popular media, but cannabis use can have permanent effects on the developing brain. The Centers for Disease Control and Prevention (CDC) notes that approximately 30% of 12th graders reported using cannabis and 6% reported using it daily in 2022.[5] So while disorder rates are relatively low, use rates are common.

Trying psychoactive substances is a common experience in adolescent development. Research has shown that many US adolescents have tried at least 1 drug before the age of 15 years, with alcohol, tobacco, and marijuana being the most common substances.[6] A key distinction between experimentation and budding dependency can be seen in whether the adolescent "craves" the substance and "needs" it to get through the day or perform daily tasks, but many teens may not be able to recognize their own loss of control over substance use.[6] Family history of addiction can also play an important role in the risk for addiction. While trying a substance may be common, it should not be "condoned, facilitated, or trivialized by adults," according to the American Academy of Pediatrics (AAP) clinical report "Substance Use Screening, Brief Intervention, and Referral to Treatment."[7] The age at first substance use is inversely correlated with the lifetime incidence of an SUD developing.[7–10]

Madison asks, "I know smoking a joint is bad for my lungs, but is vaping marijuana bad for my health? What about marijuana gummies?"

- In the short term, cannabis can have adverse effects such as increased heart rate, conjunctival injection, dry mouth, orthostatic hypotension, increased appetite, increased thirst, drowsiness, insomnia, anxiety symptoms, panic attacks, short-term memory loss, hallucinations, and ataxia.
- Youth who use cannabis are more likely than those who do not to report anxiety, existential distress, low self-esteem, and anhedonia.[4,11]
- There is also a risk for serious mental illness, including anxiety, depression, suicidality, and psychosis. It is well-documented that tetrahydrocannabinol (THC) use can induce psychosis-like symptoms (eg, cannabis-induced psychosis).[12,13] More recent research shows that frequent use and/or high doses of THC are more likely to bring on first-episode psychosis, with 2- to 5-times increased risk.[13]
- In the long term, cannabis use disrupts brain development. The brain of an adolescent is still developing until their early 20s. Cannabis negatively affects focus and motivation, reduces academic success, can affect long-term career growth, and may lower IQ.[10,13,14]

••• Communication Pearl •••
Explaining to Patients the Impact of Substance Use on the Brain

You can use a strengths-based communication approach to explain how substance use affects a patient's developing brain. For example, "By using [insert substance(s)] as a teenager, you are potentially changing your brain and not giving it the best chance to develop to reach your future goals!"

You can personalize this by talking about specific goals that the patient has mentioned.

According to the CDC, marijuana use is associated with difficulty thinking and problem-solving, reduced coordination, and difficulty maintaining attention.[5] Cannabis is an addictive substance. The earlier the age that someone begins using it, the higher their risk for addiction. Some studies show that 1 in 6 people who use cannabis (17%) become dependent when they start before age 18 years and 25% to 50% of adolescents who heavily use cannabis can become addicted.[7,8] Cannabis use accounts for the largest number of admissions for SUD treatment in publicly funded programs (76% of adolescents aged 12–17 years).[15] Tetrahydrocannabinol activates the reward system in a similar way as other addictive substances.[6,10] Additionally, although administration methods such as vaping or gummies may seem "cleaner" and appeal to youth, these methods can deliver high doses of THC, and in many cases, teens do not know what they are vaping.[16] When it comes to cannabis gummies, there is a delay in effect given the need for absorption in the body. In comparison to smoking/vaping, which can take minutes, edible THC can take 30 to 60 minutes to take effect and can be felt in the system for 3 to 4 hours post-ingestion. This delay can lead to overdosing, as adolescents, who tend to behave more impulsively because their prefrontal cortex is still developing, may think it is "not working."[13,14]

••• Communication Pearl •••
Praise the Bravery in Showing Up, Sharing, and Asking Questions

If your patient appears to engage in risk-taking behaviors or seems to ignore your advice on how to keep themselves safe and healthy but, while in clinic, is honest and asks good questions, praise them for engaging in thoughtful conversation with you. We don't often give our adolescent patients enough credit for taking these initial steps in making healthy choices. You can say, "Thank you for sharing that with me today!" or "I am so glad you felt safe telling me about that."

➤ What are common comorbidities with SUD that may co-occur with or mimic SUD that you should consider?

Excessive substance use commonly co-occurs with other mental health conditions, such as anxiety, depression, and attention-deficit/hyperactivity disorder, so it would be reasonable to consider and/or screen for those.[3,15,17] In addition, learning disabilities are associated with the increased risk of an SUD developing, so for an adolescent such as Madison, with declining grades, this diagnosis should be considered.[6,9] Unidentified learning difficulties can cause stress and frustration in school that may lead to her willingness to use cannabis as a coping mechanism for school-related stress. Similarly, anxiety and depression can interfere with social functioning, and adolescents may use substances as a social lubricant that allows them to overcome interfering symptoms.[7,9] Exposure to adverse childhood experiences (ACEs) is another risk factor for SUD developing, so considering trauma history (eg, exposure to violence, divorce) is important and may warrant screening for posttraumatic stress disorder if the onset of substance use occurred after a particularly upsetting experience.[1] Schizophrenia can be comorbid with substance use, and although rare, the onset of bipolar disorder or schizophrenia in late adolescence can occur, so screening for hallucinations, delusions, and mania should be included.[12,13] Last, drug or alcohol intoxication and withdrawal can mimic many physical illnesses and may be a medical emergency. In this case, the patient did not experience these symptoms, but for patients with underlying chronic disease, consider how drug or alcohol use may affect the management of their chronic disease.[15,18]

➤ What is your next step with Madison?

Management: Substance Use

Brief interventions: Clinicians can follow the substance use screening, brief intervention, and referral to treatment (SBIRT) framework to develop a brief intervention during visits such as this. Brief intervention strategies by use type include[7]

- **No substance use:** Provide positive reinforcement of healthy habits.
  - The NIAAA recommends including a "normative correction" statement whenever screening children or younger adolescents, such as "I am glad to hear that you, just like most others your age, have never tried alcohol."[7]
- **Substance use without an SUD:** Focus on negative health consequences and leverage personal strengths.
  - For example, "For the sake of your health, I advise you to quit smoking marijuana. Marijuana use interferes with concentration and memory and is linked to getting lower grades at school."
- **Mild to moderate SUD:** Use motivational interviewing techniques, such as Elicit-Provide-Elicit; assess stage of readiness to act; listen for and reflect "change talk"; address barriers to change.
- **Severe SUD:** Remain engaged with the family; conduct a risk assessment for harm; refer for higher levels of care.

Given that Madison has substance use that has not reached the level of diagnosable disorder, at this stage, the clinician should advise that she stop, provide counseling regarding the medical harms of marijuana use, and promote her strengths.

- For example, "Thank you so much for sharing with me about your vaping because it helps me understand more about you. You told me today about how your grades are a source of stress for you, so I'm worried your marijuana use is affecting your academic performance because marijuana can hurt your short-term memory. If your grades continue to decline, your mom might not let you continue in choir, and you are such a fantastic singer. I know singing in the choir is important to you. Do you think you might try cutting back on vaping?"

The clinician can set up a follow-up appointment with Madison to make sure her substance use has not progressed and to reward any positive changes she makes moving forward. Together they can also decide whether or not meeting with a mental health specialist would help her develop healthy coping skills and address her declining school function.

At the end of the appointment, Madison asks if you will sign her learner's permit form.

➤ What is your advice for Madison about marijuana and driving?

- To Madison: "The use of drugs can make driving a car less safe, especially when drugs are combined. The driver is more likely to weave lanes when they have used marijuana before driving. This is why driving under the influence of drugs or alcohol is illegal and can result in the loss of your license. Let's come up with a plan for how you will stop using marijuana so you can achieve your goal of getting your license and then we can see how you are doing at your follow-up appointment."

If Madison's drug use escalates to the level of being an SUD, this may need to be disclosed on her learner's permit form as a condition that would prevent control of a motor vehicle. Check state reporting guidelines about how and when to report this.

Back to the Case: Substance Use Disorder

Madison returns 6 months later with her mom, who thinks Madison's behavior has changed dramatically (she is up all night and sleeps in late, she is moody and argumentative, and she is hanging out with all-new friends). Her grades have declined and she was kicked out of choir. Madison's mom would like her to take a drug test because she's worried Madison's marijuana may be laced with something else. She's heard about fentanyl on the news and wants Madison to know if she's exposing herself to something deadly, but Madison doesn't want to take a drug test.

➤ Is drug testing a good option in this clinical setting?

While drug testing may be used in the emergency department for acute intoxication, in inpatient settings, and in drug treatment programs, it is not used routinely in the office setting or for screening purposes.[13,14] When caregivers ask about drug testing, it is important to partner with them to discuss what they hope drug testing will accomplish. Often the results of a drug test will just confirm what is already suspected, but in the process, the clinician may lose the patient's trust. Discuss with the caregiver that the patient needs to consent for drug testing in the office setting and that the results will be disclosed to the patient. In other words, the caregiver will still need to have trust and open communication with their child to learn the results of the drug test, so building this trust is our first and primary goal.[1,7] Often adolescents will want to do a drug test to prove something to their caregivers, but that is up to them and it is important to discuss the pros and cons of testing, including the possibilities that there can be false positives and that some substances, such as marijuana, can be present for up to 1 month after use.[14,15]

The SBIRT framework[7] includes providing clarity on types of treatment options, but many families underappreciate that treatment may be needed for SUD. What are some treatment options for Madison (Table 4–1)?

Table 4–1. Treatment Options for Substance Use Disorder, Including Benefits and Challenges[a]

Option	Benefits	Challenges
Individual counseling	• Empowerment and individual support to help make a change • Could help support decisions around the necessity of a higher level of care	• May lack social or family support to help maintain abstinence
Group therapy	• Social norming with peers • Cost effective	• Mixed evidence on effectiveness
Family-based therapy	• Best validated approach • Targets some of the root causes	• Time intensive for multiple family members
Intensive outpatient program	• Plethora of programs in a limited period	• Time intensive: 2–3 days per week, 9 hours per week
Partial hospitalization	• Concentrated treatment focus	• Time intensive: 5–6 days per week, 20+ hours per week

[a] A helpful website is Treatment Atlas (https://treatmentatlas.org), where you can search for addiction treatment programs near you.

➤ Are there medications that can be used to treat SUD as an outpatient?

Several additional training options are available for those interested in the treatment of SUD through a partnership between the AAP and the American Academy of Addiction Psychiatry (www.aap.org/en/patient-care/substance-use-and-prevention/training-to-treat-opioid-use-disorder-in-adolescents). Here is a list of some of the medications that may be used.

- Opioid use disorder: buprenorphine, naltrexone, methadone
- Nicotine use disorder: nicotine replacement therapy, varenicline, bupropion
- Alcohol use disorder: naltrexone, acamprosate, disulfiram
- Cannabis use disorder: *N*-acetylcysteine, topiramate

We have learned that "Just say no" is not always enough for adolescents, so it can be helpful to role-play a few other answers to resist peer pressure. The following suggestions may be useful for adolescents when they are in a situation in which they feel pressured to drink or smoke[9]:

- "I'm the designated driver—you're welcome!"
- "Addiction runs in my family."
- "I'm allergic to alcohol."
- "I'm gluten intolerant" (therefore, can't drink beer).
- "Alcohol triggers my migraines."
- "My parents give me drug tests."
- "I'm taking a medication that doesn't mix with alcohol."
- "I have an upcoming meet (eg, wrestling, track) or performance (eg, dance) and I need to be at my best."

Consider that some patients may engage in health-risk behaviors other than substance use, such as multiple sex partners and/or unprotected sex, or unregulated tattoos or piercings, or may have delayed routine medical care.[7] You should leave time for conversations regarding other health-risk behavior and may also want to do some screening laboratory tests, such as

- Complete blood cell count
- Comprehensive metabolic panel
- Hepatitis A virus (HAV) and C virus (HCV) antibodies
- Hepatitis B surface antibody (HBsAb) and surface antigen (HBsAg)
- HIV
- Syphilis
- Gonorrhea and chlamydia
- Urine pregnancy

In addition, a patient's vaccination records should be reviewed (if available) to confirm that they are up to date, including hepatitis A and B vaccines, as well as routine adolescent vaccines such as tetanus, diphtheria, acellular pertussis; meningococcal; and human papillomavirus.

Giving a prescription for naloxone to anyone at high risk for opioid exposure is good practice.[19] This includes anyone with an SUD or who lives with someone with an SUD, as well as anyone who is prescribed opioids for any reason. Fentanyl has been found in methamphetamine, cocaine, and marijuana; therefore, it is not only those with opioid use disorder who are at risk for overdose and death, as unintentional overdose is common.[19,20] While naloxone is available over the counter, cost can be a barrier.[19] There are community programs that often dispense naloxone for free, so become aware of local community groups for your patients. In many states, you can access no- or reduced-cost naloxone through NEXT Distro Naloxone (https://nextdistro.org/naloxone) and its affiliated programs.

••• Communication Pearl ••• Motivational Interviewing

Motivational interviewing skills are helpful in communicating about substance use, but a full discussion of these techniques is beyond the scope of this chapter.[21–23] Briefly, some of the principles that can be incorporated into the pediatric setting include

1. Express empathy: "It sounds like you are upset about how your relationship with your mom has changed and that has been hard on you both. It must be hard to feel like your mom does not trust you."
2. Roll with resistance: "It sounds like quitting would be challenging during finals, but we might be able to think about it when you feel less stressed. It can be frustrating to hear our concerns about this when your friends are also doing it, but there are real potential consequences that are important to think about when you're ready to hear them."
3. Explore discrepancies: "You say you could never quit, but remember that time you didn't smoke for the basketball tournament week? What made you successful that week that you could try again?"
4. Support self-efficacy: "I'm proud of you for talking with me about this and agreeing to try to make a change. It may be hard, but I believe in you and I can see you believe in yourself enough to try to make a change."

➤ Acknowledging that ACEs can be a contributing factor to an SUD developing is important, but what are some protective factors for adolescents?

In this case, Madison's religious beliefs may be protective. In addition, school connectedness and adult support are protective factors, so getting adolescents involved in clubs or sports with adult role models can be beneficial.[24,25]

Conclusion

In this case, we see the importance of the SBIRT framework being implemented in primary care. Even though the adolescent did not meet diagnostic criteria for an SUD initially, there were still ways to engage brief interventions and referrals to help with her problematic use. This case helps us recognize the context in which adolescents use substances and how we can partner with parents to keep adolescents safe. Our knowledge of the neurodevelopmental aspects of substance use and the best approaches to protect adolescents are an area of growing knowledge and active research.[17]

Lessons Learned From the Leaf

In the Leaf case (as substance use unfolds), the developing brain of an adolescent puts them at risk for both substance use and addiction to those substances.[17] In addition, there are a variety of social factors that contribute to substance use but that can also protect against problematic use and SUD. We know that supportive adults can play a protective role, and this includes health care professionals.

- Substance use disorder is a neurochemical disease. The behaviors clinicians see that can be problematic are driven by the need to fill or avoid emptying receptors that substances bind to, creating neurochemical changes. Therefore, it is important to see that SUD is a disease and not a symptom.[9,10,15]
- Confidentiality with adolescents is important, but clinicians may want to discuss involving caregivers early in conversations about SUD. Remember that caregivers must be involved in any conversation in which adolescent safety is a concern. This is an important bidirectional conversation, as it is important for the caregiver to understand and respect that the adolescent has a right to privacy and privileged content, which can be hard for caregivers to do.
- Use the SBIRT framework.[7]
- The S2BI is a helpful and quick screening tool that can be used in primary care for frequency of tobacco, alcohol, and marijuana use, in addition to other drug use if using branching logic.[2]
- Co-occurring disorders are common and should be screened for frequently throughout SUD treatment, including anxiety, depression, suicidality, and trauma.[3,15,17]
- Motivational interviewing strategies should be used in SUD counseling. Use open-ended questions, reflective listening, and empathic communication, and meet patients where they are.

Keywords: ACEs, alcohol use, cannabis use, confidentiality, motivational interviewing, nicotine use, SBIRT, substance use

Suggested Reading

Steele DW, Becker SJ, Danko KJ, et al. *Interventions for Substance Use Disorders in Adolescents: A Systematic Review*. Agency for Healthcare Research and Quality; 2020. https://www.ncbi.nlm.nih.gov/sites/books/NBK557291

References

1. Coble C, Srivastav S, Glick A, Bradshaw C, Osman C. Teaching SSHADESS versus HEADSS to medical students: an association with improved communication skills and increased psychosocial factor assessments. *Acad Pediatr*. 2023;23(1):209–215 PMID: 36130691
2. National Institute on Drug Abuse. Screening to Brief Intervention (S2BI). Accessed February 2, 2026. https://nida.nih.gov/s2bi
3. American Psychiatric Association. Cannabis use disorder. In: *Diagnostic and Statistical Manual of Mental Disorders*. 5th ed, text rev. American Psychiatric Association Publishing; 2022:575
4. Sultan RS, Zhang AW, Becker TD, et al. Cannabis use among US adolescents. *Pediatrics*. 2026;157(1):e2024070509 PMID: 41429181
5. Centers for Disease Control and Prevention. Cannabis and teens. Cannabis and Public Health. February 15, 2024. Accessed February 2, 2026. https://www.cdc.gov/cannabis/health-effects/cannabis-and-teens.html
6. Khurana A, Romer D, Betancourt LM, Brodsky NL, Giannetta JM, Hurt H. Experimentation versus progression in adolescent drug use: a test of an emerging neurobehavioral imbalance model. *Dev Psychopathol*. 2015;27(3):901–913 PMID: 25154377
7. Levy SJ, Williams JF; American Academy of Pediatrics Committee on Substance Use and Prevention. Substance use screening, brief intervention, and referral to treatment. *Pediatrics*. 2016;138(1):e20161211 PMID: 27325634
8. Hingson RW, Zha W. Age of drinking onset, alcohol use disorders, frequent heavy drinking, and unintentionally injuring oneself and others after drinking. *Pediatrics*. 2009;123(6):1477–1484 PMID: 19482757
9. Lahey J. *The Addiction Inoculation: Raising Healthy Kids in a Culture of Dependence*. Harper; 2021
10. Chambers RA, Taylor JR, Potenza MN. Developmental neurocircuitry of motivation in adolescence: a critical period of addiction vulnerability. *Am J Psychiatry*. 2003;160(6):1041–1052 PMID: 12777258
11. Gobbi G, Atkin T, Zytynski T, et al. Association of cannabis use in adolescence and risk of depression, anxiety, and suicidality in young adulthood: a systematic review and meta-analysis. *JAMA Psychiatry*. 2019;76(4):426–434 PMID: 30758486
12. Starzer MSK, Nordentoft M, Hjorthøj C. Rates and predictors of conversion to schizophrenia or bipolar disorder following substance-induced psychosis. *Am J Psychiatry*. 2018;175(4):343–350 PMID: 29179576
13. Di Forti M, Quattrone D, Freeman TP, et al; EU-GEI WP2 Group. The contribution of cannabis use to variation in the incidence of psychotic disorder across Europe (EU-GEI): a multicentre case-control study. *Lancet Psychiatry*. 2019;6(5):427–436 PMID: 30902669

14. Osterhoudt K. Edible marijuana dangers: how parents can prevent THC poisoning. HealthyChildren.org. October 11, 2023. Accessed February 3, 2026. https://www.healthychildren.org/English/ages-stages/teen/substance-abuse/Pages/Edible-Marijuana-Dangers.aspx
15. Bukstein OG, Bernet W, Arnold V, et al; Work Group on Quality Issues. Practice parameter for the assessment and treatment of children and adolescents with substance use disorders. *J Am Acad Child Adolesc Psychiatry*. 2005;44(6):609–621 PMID: 15908844
16. Chung J, Lim CCW, Stjepanović D, Hall W, Connor JP, Chan GCK. Adolescent cannabis vaping trends (2021–2023): delta-9-tetrahydrocannabinol, cannabidiol, and synthetic cannabinoids. *Am J Prev Med*. 2025;69(6):107655 PMID: 40590811
17. Nackers KAM, Kokotailo P, Levy SJL. Substance abuse, general principles. *Pediatr Rev*. 2015;36(12):535–544 PMID: 26628734
18. Vaughan BL, Knight JR. Intensive drug treatment. In: Neinstein LS, Gordon CM, Katzman DK, Rosen DS, Woods ER, eds. *Adolescent Healthcare: A Practical Guide*. 5th ed. Lippincott Williams & Wilkins; 2008:958–968
19. McKnight E, Holland-Hall C. Pediatricians' role in overdose prevention: a call for universal naloxone dispensing. *Pediatrics*. 2024;154(4):e2024067258 PMID: 39262377
20. Carney BL, Hadland SE, Bagley SM. Medication treatment of adolescent opioid use disorder in primary care. *Pediatr Rev*. 2018;39(1):43–45 PMID: 2929229
21. Erickson SJ, Gerstle M, Feldstein SW. Brief interventions and motivational interviewing with children, adolescents, and their parents in pediatric health care settings: a review. *Arch Pediatr Adolesc Med*. 2005;159(12):1173–1180 PMID: 16330743
22. McCambridge J, Slym RL, Strang J. Randomized controlled trial of motivational interviewing compared with drug information and advice for early intervention among young cannabis users. *Addiction*. 2008;103(11):1809–1818 PMID: 18778385
23. Barnes AJ, Gold MA. Promoting healthy behaviors in pediatrics: motivational interviewing. *Pediatr Rev*. 2012;33(9):e57–e68 PMID: 22942370
24. Rigg KK, Johnson ME. Preventing adolescent opioid misuse: racial/ethnic differences in the protective effects of extracurricular activities. *J Stud Alcohol Drugs*. 2022;83(3):402–411 PMID: 35590181
25. Table 3.2. In: Office of the Surgeon General, Substance Abuse and Mental Health Services Administration. *Facing Addiction in America: The Surgeon General's Report on Alcohol, Drugs, and Health*. US Dept of Health and Human Services; 2016. Accessed May 15, 2026. https://www.ncbi.nlm.nih.gov/books/NBK424850/table/ch3.t3

CHAPTER 5

Somatic Symptoms and Depression

The Butterfly: Characterized by transformation, with highs and lows, and variable abilities over time.

Presentation

Florence is a 15-year-old transgender girl who has come to your office with excessive fatigue. Their mom says Florence has been experiencing fatigue over the past 6 months, but the symptoms have worsened in the past month, causing them to sometimes be so tired that they can't get out of bed. Mom is worried because Florence has missed 5 days of school in the past 2 weeks. Florence says they are getting enough sleep (9–11 hours per night) but still feel really tired all day. There is no history of snoring, restless legs syndrome, or other sleep-related disorders. Florence's mom brought them in because Florence reported not only that they were fatigued today but that their legs felt weak. When Florence woke up, they told Mom that they couldn't stand up. Eventually, they were able to get up and walk, but Florence reports that their legs felt like they might give out and were weaker than usual. Florence says their legs look normal, and your examination confirms there is no swelling, redness, warmth, rashes, or other visible abnormalities. Florence does not remember any injuries or trauma to their legs and had a regular day yesterday. In the office, Florence has normal, stable vital signs without orthostatic changes, notable only for recent weight loss.

Patient History and Review of Systems

- **Medical history:** Gender dysphoria, migraine headaches.
- **Family history:** Mom: depression, hypothyroidism.
- **Social history:** Lives with their mom, dad, and brother. Has a pet dog. Attends a private school and is an honor student. No drugs/alcohol/smoking. Not sexually active. No history of anxiety/depression/suicidal ideation.
- **Medications:** Estradiol, Supprelin implant.
- **Gastrointestinal:** Decreased appetite, constipation.
- **Cardiovascular:** Occasional lightheadedness.
- **Neurological:** Brain fog.
- **General:** Unintentional weight loss (2 lb) over the past month.

The examination findings are normal except for concerns in the musculoskeletal and neurological evaluations.

- **Musculoskeletal:** warm and well perfused; no joint swelling or pain; full range of motion at hip, knees, and ankles; slow, cautious gait
- **Neurological:** 5/5 strength but notable for breakaway weakness; 2+ patellar reflexes; normal sensation to light touch and pinprick

There are some key questions to ask while eliciting the history that will help narrow down the differential diagnosis.[1]

- "Is there difficulty climbing stairs or combing hair?" "Do you get more tired over the day or as you exercise?"
  — These questions suggest weakness and fatiguability of a neurological etiology.
- "Do you need to stop and rest during gym class or while playing a game?"
  — This question suggests exercise intolerance, which should lead us to examine cardiac, metabolic, pulmonary, and muscle etiologies of fatigue.
- "Do you feel sleepy during the day and/or take naps? How well do you sleep at night?"
  — This question suggests a sleep-related cause and would lead toward a sleep study or ears, nose, and throat evaluation.
- "How are things going socially at school?"
  — This question suggests somatic symptom disorder or mental health issues as a possible diagnostic pathway to explore.

In summary, Florence is a 15-year-old transgender girl taking gender-affirming hormones experiencing fatigue, functional lower-extremity weakness, decreased appetite and weight loss, lightheadedness, and brain fog for the past month, with mostly normal findings on neurological examination.

➤ **Is there one diagnosis that explains Florence's symptoms, or do you think there are multiple causes for their symptoms?**

Differential Diagnosis

Florence may have an overarching diagnosis that explains this constellation of symptoms or may have multiple diagnoses that explain individual symptoms, so a multipronged approach may be indicated. The differential diagnosis is not exhaustive but represents some of the more common diagnoses to consider for this patient's history.

- **Vitamin or nutrient deficiency**
  - *Anemia:* Can cause fatigue, malaise, and lightheadedness. In this case, a history of pallor, shortness of breath, tachycardia, or blood loss is not given. Dietary intake is also unknown.
  - *Vitamin B_{12} deficiency:* Can be associated with fatigue and can cause neurological symptoms such as muscle weakness, numbness, balance issues, and paresthesia. Dietary intake is unknown, and there is no known history for why Florence would have a vitamin B_{12} deficiency, such as celiac disease, Crohn disease, thyroid disease, or use of certain medications, such as histamine blockers and proton pump inhibitors.
- **Hypothyroidism:** Symptoms include fatigue, constipation, and brain fog. Florence does not have the symptoms of cold intolerance, hair loss, dry skin, high cholesterol level, bradycardia, and weight gain.
- **Epstein-Barr virus (EBV):** Symptoms often include fatigue but also include fever, pharyngitis, enlarged lymph nodes, and rash, which they do not have. Adolescents are often symptomatic with EBV and may feel fatigued for weeks or months after the acute infection.
- **Lyme disease:** Early symptoms include a rash (erythema migrans) and flu-like symptoms (eg, headache, fatigue, swollen lymph nodes). Late-stage disease can include nerve symptoms and joint issues.
- **HIV infection:** Early symptoms of HIV infection may include flu-like symptoms including fatigue, muscle aches, weight loss, and decreased appetite. In this case, Florence responds that they are not sexually active, but adolescents do not always report sexual activity to their health care professionals.
- **Malignancy:** Symptoms include fatigue and weight loss. It is reassuring that there is no history of lymphadenopathy, easy bruising, headaches, vision changes, or respiratory distress.

- **Celiac disease:** Symptoms include fatigue, weight loss, and constipation. The symptoms of celiac disease can be vague and varied, so it is important to make sure this has been ruled out by laboratory evaluation and not symptoms alone once it is suspected.
- **Rhabdomyolysis:** Symptoms include muscle weakness and fatigue; however, it would more likely be the whole body than just lower extremities. In this case, there is no report of dark urine or oliguria and there is no preceding trauma, dehydration, infection, or excessive exercise as a potential trigger.
- **Postural orthostatic tachycardia syndrome:** Often starts around puberty and is more common in girls than boys. Symptoms can be triggered by changing from a supine to standing position. Symptoms often include palpitations, chest discomfort, lightheadedness/dizziness/fainting, exercise intolerance, and extreme fatigue. In this case, there is no history of orthostatic symptoms/signs or cardiac symptoms, but there are reports of fatigue and lightheadedness.
- **Depression:** The symptoms of depression that are seen in this case include poor sleep with daytime somnolence, acute change in school attendance, and, possibly, psychomotor retardation.
- **Somatic symptom and related disorders (SSRD):** In the *Diagnostic and Statistical Manual of Mental Disorders, Fifth Edition, Text Revision* (*DSM-5-TR*), this is an umbrella term for a variety of conditions including functional neurological disorders and disorders of gut-brain interaction. Somatic symptom and related disorders are caused by disruptions in mind-body connections, and a diagnosis is made when one or more somatic symptoms cause distress or significantly disrupt daily life and the patient has excessive thoughts, feelings, or behaviors related to the somatic symptoms over a period of 6 months.[2]

Keep in Mind: Diagnosis of Inclusion

Somatic symptom and related disorders are not a diagnosis of exclusion. Patients can be given this diagnosis while undergoing a workup for additional organic etiologies of their symptoms. This has been called the "walking 2 paths" philosophy, in which somatic symptoms are treated simultaneously with an evaluation for organic pathology.[3]

A helpful clinical pathway for SSRD can be found online (www.chop.edu/clinical-pathway/somatic-symptom-related-disorders-ssrd-clinical-pathway).

Evaluation

To evaluate a patient for fatigue, consider the following laboratory tests:

- Complete blood cell count
- Iron studies
- Thyrotropin (previously referred to as *thyroid-stimulating hormone*) function
- Vitamin B_{12} level
- Epstein-Barr virus serology

The following additional tests may also be useful in the evaluation:

- C-reactive protein level
- Erythrocyte sedimentation rate
- Comprehensive metabolic panel
- Celiac disease panel
- Creatine phosphokinase level
- Enzyme-linked immunosorbent assay (ELISA) and Western blot tests for Lyme disease

When evaluating a patient for SSRD, a few additional history questions that may be helpful to better define an illness timeline, potential triggering events, patient goals, and barriers to functioning include

- When was the last time you felt completely healthy?
- What are your top 3 disabling symptoms?
- Which of your symptoms keep you from doing what you want to be doing?

Simultaneously, screening for any mental health issues, particularly depression, is appropriate, considering that Florence has had poor sleep, decreased school attendance, and psychomotor retardation, which are seen in patients with depression.

The following validated screening tools are used widely in clinical practice. Refer to the Appendix for links to the tools online.

- **Pediatric Symptom Checklist-17 (PSC-17):** Widely used parent-completed measure of a child's psychosocial functioning, normed for children and adolescents aged 4 to 17 years, including internalized problems (eg, anxiety, depression), attention issues, and externalizing problems (eg, disruptive and oppositional behaviors). This is a briefer version of the PSC-35.
    - A score of 15 or higher suggests the need for further follow-up and an evaluation for the presence of a mental health disorder. Similarly, each subscale has a cutoff score.
        - Attention—7
        - Externalizing—7
        - Internalizing—5

- **Patient Health Questionnaire-9 Modified for Adolescents (PHQ-A):** A depression and suicidality screening tool for youth aged 11 to 17 years. The PHQ-A consists of 8 items that help classify differences in levels of depressive symptoms and 1 item related to suicidal ideation (eg, "Thoughts that you would be better off dead, or of hurting yourself in some way?"). It can be a helpful tool when assessing for anxiety, as the 2 disorders are highly comorbid. It can also serve as a symptom tracker and progress-monitoring tool if used over time.
  - Cutoff scores are
    - 5—mild
    - 10—moderate
    - 15—moderately severe
    - 20—severe
  - If suicidal ideation is endorsed, it requires immediate follow-up with a more investigative suicide screener, such as the Ask Suicide-Screening Questions (ASQ) or Columbia-Suicide Severity Rating Scale (C-SSRS); safety planning; and referral for external support. Refer to Chapter 9, Suicidality and Eating Disorder, for further discussion on suicidality.
- **Strengths and Difficulties Questionnaire (SDQ):** A general behavioral screening questionnaire, normed for children and adolescents aged 2 to 17 years, that focuses on emotional symptoms, conduct, hyperactivity/impulsivity, peer relationships, and prosocial behavioral concerns. The questionnaire does not follow diagnostic criteria as the former 2 questionnaires do but can flag areas of concern and prosocial strengths.
  - 25 items; can be completed by parents, teachers, or child (age dependent)
- **Ask Suicide-Screening Questions (ASQ):** Suicide risk screening tool; validated for youth 10 years and older but can be used for children as young as 8 years.
  - 4 questions; a response of "Yes" to at least 1 is identified as a suicide risk.
  - The American Academy of Pediatrics (AAP) recommends universal suicide screening for youth 12 years and older.

Back to the Case: Somatic Symptom Disorder

The results of Florence's laboratory tests were normal. In the week since being seen in clinic, Florence continued to have intermittent lower-extremity weakness followed by periods of normal functioning. Florence has been using a wheelchair to navigate school because of their weakness but has been able to ambulate up the stairs in their 2-story home. Florence has some lightheadedness but no dizziness, headaches, syncope, or vision changes. Florence's mom reports that they are eating well but could improve hydration.

Back to the Case (*continued*)

Florence completed the PHQ-A and had a score of 5, which is consistent with mild depression. They had no suicidal thoughts or behaviors. Florence endorsed feeling somewhat hopeless, as if this is just their life and they must get used to unexplainable pain and discomfort. Florence has been missing some days of school because of their symptoms, and Florence's mom is upset that no one seems to know what is wrong and Florence isn't getting better.

➤ Is any further evaluation needed to make the diagnosis of somatic symptom disorder?

The diagnosis of somatic symptom disorder is a clinical one, so no further laboratory tests or imaging is needed. This is now at the top of our differential diagnosis list given the following findings:

- Inconsistency and variability in symptoms
- Symptoms that depend on context (ie, needing a wheelchair at school but not at home)
- Physical exam findings inconsistent with reported symptoms (ie, 5/5 strength in lower extremities with reported ability to climb stairs)

While the workup of other pathologies may be pursued ("walking 2 paths"), your confidence in this diagnosis should be expressed to the patient and family.[1,3] Engaging in shared decision-making about the limited efficacy of performing additional tests or studies given the likely diagnosis of somatic symptom disorder can help build rapport and demonstrate support of patients and families that have been searching for a diagnosis.

Discussion: Somatic Symptom Disorder

Children and adolescents with somatic symptom disorder are often over-medicalized and receive excessive evaluations of their symptoms, including laboratory tests, imaging, and multiple specialty referrals.[3] It is difficult for caregivers to see their child physically struggling when there does not appear to be a direct cause or trauma to the body. Helping caregivers connect a physical symptom with a mental health diagnosis can be challenging and requires sensitivity and patience.

In conveying this diagnosis to caregivers and adolescents, it is important that clinicians not only offer the diagnosis but explain it, as the diagnosis itself sounds like jargon. Also, because the patient may have already been through a few rounds of tests and they and their family may be frustrated by the lack of diagnosis, there may be an emotional response to the diagnosis for which the clinician should be prepared to respond.[3]

In delivering this diagnosis, the clinician should name it and explain it, as shown in the following example:

- I know what is causing Florence's symptoms. Florence has somatic symptom disorder, which means their symptoms are caused by a problem in how their mind and body are communicating.

It is important that all health care team members provide consistent messaging and terminology, as any uncertainty expressed by health care professionals can lead patients to lose trust in their own diagnosis and treatment plan.

Consider that culture and context inform how patients and families may receive the diagnosis.[4,5] The mind-body framework can carry stigma and may not be accepted by everyone. Alternative explanations (eg, "nervous system and body") may be a better fit for an individual patient/family.[3]

••• Communication Pearl •••
Normalizing Somatization

Everyone has experienced somatic symptoms. Think about a time when you were nervous, and you felt butterflies in your stomach—those are somatic symptoms. Most of the time, these symptoms are harmless and short-lived, but for some children and adolescents, these become amplified and may interfere with daily life.

Resources for communicating about the diagnosis of SSRD and a potential clinical pathway can be found online.

- Communication Tips (www.chop.edu/clinical-pathway/somatic-symptom-related-disorders-ssrd-communication-tips)
- Emergency Department and Inpatient Clinical Pathway for Somatic Symptoms and Related Disorders (www.chop.edu/clinical-pathway/somatic-symptom-related-disorders-ssrd-clinical-pathway)

It is important to let the family know that there are treatment pathways that will help Florence, but they take time and dedication.

➤ Are there coexisting conditions that are common with SSRD?

Somatic symptom and related disorders are associated with other mental health disorders, particularly anxiety and depression, which each occur in up to 50% of patients and contribute to the interference with functioning and cause distress.[6] Other mental health disorders to consider include posttraumatic stress disorder and obsessive-compulsive disorder.

There are also risk factors for SSRD that should be considered, including adverse childhood experiences (eg, exposure to sexual trauma, intimate partner violence, and abuse).[2] These may coexist and require separate assessment, intervention, or management.

Keep in Mind: Gender-Affirming Care

Transgender patients may seem to be overrepresented in mental health care. Many studies have demonstrated that transgender adolescents face high rates of internalizing psychopathology, likely caused by the stress of experiencing discrimination, stigma, bullying, and lack of acceptance by peers and family.[7,8] Family nonacceptance has been found to be a significant correlate of suicidality.[7,8] However, take special care to not assume that any mental health issues are related to gender dysphoria, and always find ways to empathetically support patients' speaking about their own experiences.[7]

A few gender-affirming strategies to implement in practice include

- Validate LGBTQIA+ identities and ask about pronouns.
- Communicate limits of confidentiality.
- Use LGBTQIA+ badge buddies with clinician pronouns.
- Seek training and education in gender-affirming care for all staff.

➤ **What treatment plan do you recommend for Florence?**

Management: Somatic Symptom Disorder

Treatment includes a combination of medical and behavioral management.[3] Physical therapy and occupational therapy can be helpful to reduce somatic symptoms, especially related to mobility, strength, function, and activities of daily living.[4] Accommodations may need to be made temporarily at school, so health care professionals can provide education not only for the family but for the school as well.[3] These accommodations should be time limited and discontinued as soon as function returns so the body can relearn these skills.[4]

While SSRD can typically be managed with outpatient primary care, some patients may need specialty referral, particularly if there are debilitating symptoms, including

- Widespread pain: Refer to an amplified pain program or rheumatologist.
- Recurrent abdominal pain: Refer to an interdisciplinary gastroenterology program that includes psychologists.

- Dizziness, presyncope: Refer to a dysautonomia program, which may include general pediatricians, rheumatologists, and/or cardiologists.
- Functional neurological disorder: Refer to a neurology or physical medicine and rehabilitation program.

Cognitive behavioral therapy is a cornerstone of treatment, as it is helpful for symptom management, stress reduction, and management of coexisting conditions, such as anxiety or depression, if they exist.[3,6] This therapy for SSRD can be explained to patients and families as "physical therapy for the brain."[4] Medication management does not tend to be helpful.[3]

Interdisciplinary communication is key. Collaboration and communication between the pediatric clinician(s), mental health specialist, physical therapist, and/or occupational therapist can help ensure that treatment goals are aligned.[3]

Back to the Case: Depression

Florence returns 6 months later. They now have a good understanding of somatic symptom disorder and, having completed their treatment course with physical therapy, feel symptom-free. Florence feels that this period was difficult socially because they lost many friends who didn't understand what they were going through. Florence couldn't participate in volleyball this year, which was their usual social and physical outlet, so now they have been more sedentary and spending more time alone in their room after school. Florence says they feel sluggish, like they're moving underwater. Florence also says they are on their phone almost constantly and find themselves crying often for almost no reason. Florence's mom says she has noted that Florence has a poor appetite and she must force them to join the family for dinner. Florence stays up until 2:00 am because they have a hard time falling asleep and then feel tired throughout the school day.

➤ What is the next step in Florence's management plan?

Continuity of care is the hallmark of pediatric care, as you can repeatedly reassess for ongoing issues. For example, because you had screened Florence for depression with the PHQ-A in the prior visit, you can readminister the screening for comparison. At this visit, Florence scores a 16, which indicates moderately severe depressive symptoms, necessitating further screening for depression and suicidality. Areas for assessment include

- Risk for suicidality or homicidality
- Psychiatric review of systems
- Mental health treatment history
- Psychosocial history
- Family medical and psychiatric history
- Academic history
- Level of functioning, impairment, and distress

After further clinical history and assessment, you learn that Florence has displayed depressed mood and loss of interest in activities (anhedonia) for more than 2 weeks. They also endorsed insomnia, psychomotor retardation, fatigue, and poor appetite (for *DSM-5-TR* diagnostic criteria, there must be ≥4 symptoms endorsed in addition to depressed mood/loss of interest or pleasure; other possible symptoms could have included weight loss or appetite change, feelings of worthlessness or guilt, difficulty concentrating, or suicidal ideation).[9] Taken together, these symptoms, along with the PHQ-A screening tool, changes in social functioning and recreational activities, and clinical assessment, meet the criteria for major depressive disorder.

➤ Who should be screened for depression?

Youth aged 12 to 18 years should be screened annually for depression with a validated screening tool, such as the PHQ-A.[6,10,11] Children younger than 12 years may not receive routine screening; however, they may benefit from screening if there are risk factors present.[6] Depression can be classified as mild, moderate, and severe, according to the *DSM-5-TR*.[9]

- Mild
  - 5 to 7 criteria in the *DSM-5-TR* for depression
  - Minor functional impairment and distress
  - No comorbid psychiatric diagnoses, psychotic symptoms (eg, delusions and/or hallucinations), or suicidal ideation
- Moderate
  - 5 to 7 criteria in the *DSM-5-TR* for depression
  - Moderate functional impairment and distress
  - No psychotic features
  - Can include comorbid psychiatric diagnoses and/or suicidal ideation
- Severe
  - At least 7 criteria in the *DSM-5-TR* for depression
  - Markedly impaired function or severe distress
  - At least 1 of the following findings: comorbid psychiatric diagnosis, suicidal ideation/behavior, depression-congruent psychotic features[9]

➤ How do you assess the patient's level of functioning, impairment, and distress?

Determining the level of functioning, impairment, and distress helps you make the diagnosis and determine its severity. During the clinical interview, you can ask about the patient's ability to interact with others, manage their daily tasks, function at school, and achieve their usual daily goals. Example questions include

- How much is your sleepiness getting in the way of you being successful at school?
- How often are you feeling like this? Is it daily?

Functioning can also be assessed by using validated instruments such as the Children's Global Assessment Scale (CGAS) and the Columbia Impairment Scale (CIS). Refer to the Appendix for links to the tools online. The CGAS is a clinician-based score of overall global psychosocial functioning on a scale of 1 to 100. It is used often in research and less in clinical practice but could still give a subjective measure of overall functioning and show areas in which further assessment or intervention is warranted.

Keep in Mind: Screening Versus Diagnosis

Many of the tools discussed are meant to screen patients for symptoms that have not yet reached the level of a diagnosable disorder. The intention is to identify those who need further evaluation for intervention. However, it is important to remember that screening tools do not determine a mental health diagnosis on their own. Be sure to understand full criteria before providing a diagnosis or refer to/consult with a mental health specialist for a full evaluation if needed.

For patients at risk for a diagnosis of depression, a helpful potential clinical pathway can be found online (www.chop.edu/clinical-pathway/depression-clinical-pathway).

Florence's mom now recalls that Florence's aunt has a diagnosis of bipolar disorder. Mom is worried because she remembers that when her sister was diagnosed, she was staying up late at night and Florence has also been up until 2:00 am every night. She asks if Florence could have the same disorder.

➤ How do you screen for psychosis and mania in patients with depression?

Psychosis and mania/hypomania can both mimic or co-occur with depression.[9] It is important to screen for these symptoms while eliciting the history, as patients may not disclose that they are having these symptoms. Some suggested questions include

- Do you ever feel your ears or eyes play tricks on you?
- Do you hear voices talking to you when no one is there?
- Does your mind ever feel confused?
- Do you ever feel like people are out to get you or like everyone is against you?
- Do people ever tell you that your moods change quickly?
- Do people ever tell you that you talk too much or too fast?
- Do you ever have bursts of energy where you stay up all night doing things?
- Has your family said that your personality changed recently?
- Do you ever have so much energy that you don't need to sleep?

After talking more with Florence, it seems they do not have any symptoms of psychosis or mania, so you can explain to their mom that their sleep disturbance is more likely related to depression than bipolar disorder. It's important, though, that Florence's mom continue to monitor for these symptoms and let you know if anything changes. It is also important to thank her for telling you that information, as having a better understanding of family history of mental health issues is important.

Keep in Mind: Suicide Screening

Screen all adolescents for suicidality, but those with depression are at higher risk for suicidal thoughts and behaviors, so this should consistently be a part of any depression evaluation.[6,11,12] Although the PHQ-A includes questions on suicidality, it is helpful to ask specific questions about suicidal ideation.

To begin the conversation, clinicians can say, "Part of my job is to ask tough questions to make sure you are safe. Is it OK if I ask you some questions about your mood?"

- Are there times when you feel sad?
- Have you ever felt so sad that you felt like life was worthless or not worth living?
- Have you ever felt so sad that you wanted to do something to take away or end the pain, such as hurting yourself or even killing yourself?
- Have you ever felt so sad that you wanted to hurt someone else?

If a patient has suicidal thoughts or behaviors, safety planning is the crucial next step. It is important to remain calm and neutral. The clinician will want to consider thanking the patient for sharing something very private or difficult and let them know they are here to support them.

The AAP has resources for conducting a brief suicide safety assessment on its website (www.aap.org/en/patient-care/blueprint-for-youth-suicide-prevention/strategies-for-clinical-settings-for-youth-suicide-prevention/conducting-a-brief-suicide-safety-assessment). The goal is to develop a safety plan before patients are in a crisis. Clinicians can rehearse strategies that patients can use for coping, as well as identify people and places that can offer help.[6,11] An important point to review with caregivers is making the environment safe. Depending on the patient and household, this may include locking up medications, safely storing firearms, and/or removing knives or ropes. During safety planning, clinicians may identify and help mitigate potential risk factors for depression and suicide, such as psychosocial stressors (eg, peer or relationship issues, bullying, bereavement).[5,6] If the patient has suicidal ideation, do not leave them unattended until next steps are determined and appropriate action is taken to guarantee their safety. Refer to Chapter 9, Suicidality and Eating Disorder, for more information about suicide and suicide prevention.

After your clinical interview and reviewing the PHQ-A with Florence and their mother, you discuss depression and major depressive disorder. Next, you will want to ask them if you can discuss resources and referrals. Although many therapeutic treatments can have a positive effect on mental health, the 3 most recommended types of psychotherapy for depression in adolescents are cognitive behavioral therapy (CBT), interpersonal psychotherapy for adolescents (IPT-A), and dialectical behavior therapy (DBT).[6,11]

Brief interventions: There are a few brief interventions for depression that can be introduced in the office setting.

- **Promotion of healthy habits**
  - Encourage your patient to stay focused on the basics: eating, sleeping, and activity.
    - Nutrition—3 healthy meals and 2 healthy snacks, with adequate water intake and reduced caffeine and sugary drinks
    - Sleep hygiene—healthy sleep habits; consistent bedtime and wake times every day of the week; reduced or ceased daytime napping; using the bed only for sleep; reduction of electronics before sleep
    - Activity—a daily goal of moving the body (eg, taking a short walk, going outside in the morning, playing with the dog)
- **Cognitive restructuring,** defined as changing unhelpful thoughts to helpful ones
  - Explain that thoughts can be like traffic lights, in which negative thoughts are red lights and helpful thoughts are green lights. When your patient identifies a red thought, such as "I'm so stupid—why do I even go to school?" they will want to immediately pause and replace that thought with a green one, such as "I enjoy my teachers, and I really like art." The thought does not have to be the most positive opposite of the negative thought (eg, "I'm the smartest in my class") but rather can be in the positive direction (eg, "I try hard at school, and I like seeing my friends").
- **Behavioral activation**
  - The goal is to help your patient in identifying rewarding or enjoyable activities to help reduce their anhedonia/avoidance behaviors and subsequently devise strategies to enhance their motivation to complete them.
  - Examples include going on a walk with a friend to get ice cream once this week, spending phone-free time with the family during dinnertime, or baking cookies—small goals that can be worked into a daily schedule.
  - In addition to performing the activity, pairing it with a reflective exercise is recommended, such as journaling or creating a mood log to help keep track of how the activities affect their mood.

Keep in Mind: Therapy Options

When recommending therapy to a patient, often the lack of specificity about what criteria to look for when seeking a therapist can contribute to barriers of care. Consider naming the type of evidence-based therapy recommended for the patient (eg, CBT, DBT), as they will have a better chance of finding the most effective treatment option for their diagnosis and likely build trust in the therapeutic process.

Conclusion

In this case, the evolving symptoms of depression are seen overlapping with the existing diagnosis of somatic symptom disorder. This highlights the importance of continuing to screen for depression with a tool such as the PHQ-A or a similar questionnaire in the setting of risk factors and a diagnosis for which there is a high comorbidity rate of anxiety and depression. Refer to Chapter 11, Depression and Depressive Disorder, for more information.

Lessons Learned From the Butterfly

In the Butterfly case (as somatic symptoms and depression unfold), the youth's journey is one of transformation, but they do not typically perceive the transformative process when they are in it. It is only in retrospect that the full journey is appreciated. During low moments, it can be challenging for a patient to see the potential for a bright future, but with positive role models supporting them, behavioral activation strategies, and close follow-up by the clinician, small iterative changes can allow the patient to successfully complete their metamorphosis.

- Patients with SSRD can "walk 2 paths," meaning that clinicians can diagnose and treat SSRD while pursuing other diagnoses.[2–4]
- Patients with SSRD are often overmedicalized. The best approach is often doing less laboratory tests, imaging, and specialty referrals. Empathic and clear communication that discusses the mind-body connection is important.[3–5]
- Anxiety and depression are common in patients with SSRD.[9]
- Depression screening should be conducted at regular intervals with a tool such as the PHQ-A to monitor depressive symptoms and suicidality over time.[6,10–12]
- Suicide screening should be done annually for all patients 12 years and older and for all patients with depression. If present, safety planning is paramount and should be done to mitigate risk factors and identify resources immediately.[5,6,11,12]
- Depression can be classified as mild, moderate, or severe, and a proper assessment along with an evaluation of functional impairment and distress will help the clinician determine the management and treatment plan, as well as the appropriate level of care.[6,9]
- There are a few brief behavioral interventions the clinician can use to help move the needle on depressive symptoms while patients wait for treatment.[6,11]

Keywords: depression, gender-affirming care, gender dysphoria, safety planning, somatic symptom and related disorder, suicide

Suggested Reading

Benton T, Staab J, Evans DL. Medical co-morbidity in depressive disorders. *Ann Clin Psychiatry.* 2007;19(4):289–303 PMID: 18058286

Rafferty J; American Academy of Pediatrics Committee on Psychosocial Aspects of Child and Family Health; Committee on Adolescence; and Section on Lesbian, Gay, Bisexual, and Transgender Health and Wellness. Ensuring comprehensive care and support for transgender and gender-diverse children and adolescents. *Pediatrics.* 2018;142(4):e20182162 PMID: 30224363

References

1. De Nardi L, Lanzetta MA, Ghirigato E, Barbi E, Gortani G. Approach to the child with fatigue: a focus for the general pediatrician. *Front Pediatr.* 2022;10:1044170 PMID: 36533226
2. American Psychiatric Association. Somatic symptom and related disorders. In: *Diagnostic and Statistical Manual of Mental Disorders.* 5th ed, text rev. American Psychiatric Association Publishing; 2022:349–370
3. Ibeziako P, Brahmbhatt K, Chapman A, et al. Developing a clinical pathway for somatic symptom and related disorders in pediatric hospital settings. *Hosp Pediatr.* 2019;9(3):147–155 PMID: 30782623
4. Wiggins A, Raniti M, Gaafar D, Court A, Sawyer SM. Pediatric somatic symptom and related disorders: parent acceptance influences recovery. *J Pediatr.* 2022;241:109–114 PMID: 34624318
5. Alegria M, Atkins M, Farmer E, Slaton E, Stelk W. One size does not fit all: taking diversity, culture and context seriously. *Adm Policy Ment Health.* 2010;37(1–2):48–60 PMID: 20165910
6. Boyd RC, Lewis J, Borreggine K, Benton T. Adolescent depression: identification and treatment. *Curr Treat Options Pediatr.* 2018;4:350–362
7. Acosta W, Qayyum Z, Turban JL, van Schalkwyk GI. Identify, engage, understand: supporting transgender youth in an inpatient psychiatric hospital. *Psychiatr Q.* 2019;90(3):601–612 PMID: 31209713
8. Seager van Dyk I, Sena R, McCord C, Kodish T, DeAntonio M. Affirming LGBTQIA+ youth in inpatient psychiatric settings. *J Am Acad Child Adolesc Psychiatry.* 2024;63(3):296–300 PMID: 37451313
9. American Psychiatric Association. Major depressive disorder. In: *Diagnostic and Statistical Manual of Mental Disorders.* 5th ed, text rev. American Psychiatric Association Publishing; 2022:184–193
10. Sun Y, Kong Z, Song Y, Liu J, Wang X. The validity and reliability of the PHQ-A on screening of depression in neurology: a cross sectional study. *BMC Psychiatry.* 2022;22(1):98 PMID: 35139810
11. Zuckerbrot RA, Cheung A, Jensen PS, Stein REK, Laraque D; GLAD-PC Steering Group. Guidelines for Adolescent Depression in Primary Care (GLAD-PC), I: practice preparation, identification, assessment, and initial management. *Pediatrics.* 2018;141(3):e20174081 PMID: 29483200
12. Hua LL, Lee J, Rahmandar MH, Sigel EJ; American Academy of Pediatrics Committee on Adolescence and Council on Injury, Violence, and Poison Prevention. Suicide and suicide risk in adolescents. *Pediatrics.* 2024;153(1):e2023064800 PMID: 38073403

CHAPTER 6

Depression of Chronic Disease

The Rain Cloud: Characterized by darkness, crying, or gloom. Look out for low energy, lack of interest, and sadness.

Presentation

London is a 12-year-old with a history of inflammatory bowel disease (IBD). She was diagnosed after a prior pediatrician noted weight loss, fatigue, and blood in her stools and is now following up with a gastroenterologist and nutritionist. She has had frequent admissions to the hospital over the past year for flares of her IBD, and during her most recent admission, she was diagnosed with malnutrition, so a nasogastric (NG) tube was placed to help supplement her caloric intake. Her dad brought her to the office today because he has noted that over the past 2 months, her mood has changed. He initially felt that she was just a "typical moody tween" and that her fatigue was related to her IBD. However, in the past month, he has found her crying in her room on a few occasions. He says she has been writing sad poems about dying that have concerned her teacher. Since her diagnosis, she has not been socializing with friends as much because she is afraid that she will have diarrhea while she is out of the house, and she is embarrassed about her NG tube. She is often late to school because she experiences symptoms in the morning while getting ready, and she is worried about her grades. She quit playing the flute because she didn't want to stay for after-school rehearsals.

➤ What additional questions do you have about London?

Because you are seeing her for the first time, you will want to elicit a full history, including family history, social history, and medications, as well as conduct a review of systems.

Patient History and Review of Systems

- **Birth history:** Born at full term.
- **Medical history:** IBD diagnosed 1 year ago. Previously healthy except for seasonal allergies. Met all developmental milestones on time.
- **Family history:** Mom with celiac disease. Paternal aunt with depression. Maternal uncle with type 1 diabetes.
- **Social history:** Lives with biological parents and 2 siblings. She is in sixth grade and is typically a high-performing student. She enjoys writing and playing the flute. She has a core group of 3 friends, whom she has known since kindergarten. She has a dog that she loves.
- **Trauma:** None known.
- **Medications:** Infliximab (Remicade), probiotic, ferrous sulfate.
- **Constitutional:** Mild fatigue.
- **Gastrointestinal:** Intermittent nausea and crampy abdominal pain.
- **Diet:** Peptamen by NG tube in 3 bolus feedings per day and by mouth at liberty as tolerated. Takes approximately 75% of calories by NG feedings.

In this case, there is a known diagnosis of IBD; however, there are new symptoms of fatigue, increased crying, and social withdrawal.

➤ How can you determine if London's symptoms are related to her primary diagnosis of IBD, are a new diagnosis, or both?

Differential Diagnosis

- **IBD flares:** A chronic, relapsing course is common with IBD, and if London's medication regimen is new, she may not yet be in remission. Inflammatory bowel disease flares can include intermittent nausea, crampy abdominal pain, mild fatigue, and decreased energy. Given that her current gastrointestinal symptoms are milder than previous episodes and her dad is reporting concerns related to her mood, this is less likely.

- **Heart failure:** Remicade has been associated with heart failure, which can present with fatigue, but she has no symptoms of shortness of breath or edema and no underlying history of heart disease.[1]
- **Nutritional deficiency:** Patients with IBD are at risk for deficiencies in iron, vitamin B_{12}, calcium, and vitamin D. Nutritional deficiencies can be associated with fatigue and changes in mood.[2–4] This patient is receiving an elemental formula and iron supplementation, and her gastrointestinal symptoms have been present for 6 months while she was being monitored by a nutritionist, making this less likely as a source of her symptoms.
  — *Iron deficiency anemia:* Although she is taking iron supplementation orally, intravenous iron is sometimes needed in patients with IBD. Iron deficiency anemia can cause fatigue and mood changes, so it should be considered in this patient.[2–4]
  — *Malnutrition:* Patients with IBD are at risk for malnutrition through a variety of mechanisms, including impaired nutrient absorption, chronic diarrhea, poor oral intake, increased nutrient needs, bacterial overgrowth, or medication adverse effects.[2,3]
- **Thyroid disease:** London has a family history of autoimmune conditions (ie, type 1 diabetes, celiac disease), as well as her personal history of IBD. She has symptoms of fatigue, weight loss, and mood swings.
- **Celiac disease:** London is at higher risk for other autoimmune conditions given her family and personal histories. Celiac disease can be more difficult to recognize in the setting of IBD because of overlapping symptoms of abdominal pain/discomfort, diarrhea, and weight loss.
- **Sleep disorder:** Patients with chronic pain and diarrhea may experience disrupted sleep because of these symptoms, which could contribute to daytime fatigue and mood changes.
- **Depression:** Patients with chronic diseases are at risk for depression, related to chronic pain, fatigue, and frustration with how the disease interferes with daily life and functioning.[2]
- **Premenstrual dysphoric disorder:** Characterized by depressed or dysphoric mood in the week before menses that improves within a few days after the onset of menses. Timing of symptoms should be tracked with menses to make the diagnosis.
- **Adjustment disorder[5]:** Depressed mood, anxiety, or behavioral difficulties in response to a stressor, such as a new IBD diagnosis, that do not meet criteria for other major mental health disorders but still interfere with daily functioning. Patients with this disorder can report a sense of incompetence, one of helplessness, one of hopelessness, and/or a desire to give up but are sometimes able to experience moments of happiness and enjoy previously pleasurable activities.
- **Social anxiety:** A reluctance to leave the house and spend time with peers may be a sign of social anxiety. This represents a change from London's baseline behavior.

- **Medication-induced emotional dysregulation:** Some medications may cause symptoms of irritability, anxiety, depression, anhedonia, emotional flattening, or aggression. The types of medications most often associated with this dysregulation are corticosteroids (used for IBD flares), antidepressants, antipsychotics, stimulants, benzodiazepines, β-blockers, anticonvulsants, opioid pain medications, hormonal medications, cytotoxic drugs (including methotrexate, used in IBD management), interferons, antihypertensives, and isotretinoin.[2,4,6] Eliciting a comprehensive medication history is therefore important. In this case, London is not currently taking any of these medications but may have been taking corticosteroids during her multiple hospital admissions.
- **Bullying:** London may be experiencing bullying at school because of her medical issues and NG tube, as her appearance has changed.

Evaluation

The first step is talking with London. It will be important for the clinician to build rapport with her, since they have not had an ongoing relationship, and she may be reluctant to open up about her symptoms given her reported social isolation, depressed mood, and emotional lability.

Include her father in the discussion to better assess how well she is engaging in activities of daily living, such as bathing, maintaining hygiene, eating meals, and doing chores. Her adherence with her IBD treatment plan can also be assessed. The conversation could include questions such as

- Is she attending appointments?
- Is she forgetting to take medications?
- Is she using her NG tube as recommended?
- Does she see a mental health specialist in gastroenterology or within her community, such as a pediatric psychologist or clinical social worker?

Caregivers can provide varying levels of autonomy to preadolescents in the management of their chronic disease. Some caregivers will begin to give their child more autonomy, while others might take on an overbearing role, so it is important to understand how much London's parents are monitoring her management and offer guidance on what they should be looking out for and reporting back to the clinician.

The clinician may want to reach out to her gastroenterologist to determine if any of her symptoms could be caused by her IBD or be potential complications of her medications and nutritional management. If a registered dietician is involved in her care, they can also be a person to consult with for further information.

To narrow down the differential diagnosis, the clinician may want to screen the patient with the following tests:

- Thyrotropin (previously referred to as *thyroid-stimulating hormone*) level, free thyroxine level
- Celiac disease panel
- Complete blood cell count; iron panel, including ferritin level
- 25-Hydroxyvitamin D
- C-reactive protein level and erythrocyte sedimentation rate
- Fecal calprotectin level

Keep in Mind: Use Clinic Mental Health Resources

Some pediatric clinicians have embedded mental health specialists within their clinic, such as pediatric psychologists or clinical social workers. These specialists are trained specifically to help patients manage the potential burden of chronic illness, including treatment adherence, emotional dysregulation or mood changes, and disease management.

Additionally, the patient should be screened for anxiety, depression, and suicide, as her father has reported concerns about her emotional state. Refer to the Appendix for links to the following tools online:

- **Screen for Child Anxiety and Related Emotional Disorders (SCARED):** A pediatric anxiety screener used for children 8 years and older. A total score of 25 or higher may indicate the presence of an anxiety disorder. Child and parent rating scale versions are available.
  - Additionally, this screener will give the clinician subscale scores, which may indicate a specific type of anxiety disorder such as generalized anxiety disorder, social anxiety disorder, panic, school anxiety, and separation anxiety.
- **Patient Health Questionnaire-9 Modified for Adolescents (PHQ-A):** A depression and suicidality screening tool for youth aged 11 to 17 years. The PHQ-A consists of 8 items that help classify differences in levels of depressive symptoms and 1 item related to suicidal ideation (eg, "Thoughts that you would be better off dead, or of hurting yourself in some way?"). It can be a helpful tool when assessing for anxiety, as the 2 disorders are highly comorbid. It can also serve as a symptom tracker and progress-monitoring tool if used over time.
  - Cutoff scores are
    - 5—mild
    - 10—moderate
    - 15—moderately severe
    - 20—severe
  - If suicidal ideation is endorsed, it requires immediate follow-up with a more investigative suicide screener, such as the Ask Suicide-Screening Questions (ASQ) or Columbia-Suicide Severity Rating Scale (C-SSRS); safety planning; and referral for external support. Refer to Chapter 9, Suicidality and Eating Disorder, for further discussion on suicidality.

- **Ask Suicide-Screening Questions (ASQ):** Suicide risk screening tool; validated for youth 10 years and older but can be used for children as young as 8 years.
  - 4 questions; a response of "Yes" to at least 1 is identified as a suicide risk.
  - The American Academy of Pediatrics (AAP) recommends universal suicide screening for youth 12 years and older.

Back to the Case: Potential Adjustment Disorder

London reports to you, "I can't go anywhere because I might have diarrhea and that would ruin my life!" When you suggest that she invite her friends over, she says, "I'm too tired to have anyone over, and there is no way I could clean my room for guests because I have no energy." Even after you say that her friends probably don't care about her messy room, she cries, "Why put them through being my friend when I'm probably going to die."

Discussion: Potential Adjustment Disorder

A low mood does not always equate with clinical depression. A person with major depressive disorder (MDD) must show depressed or irritable mood or markedly diminished interest or pleasure in activities for most of the day, nearly every day over a 2-week period, that is a change from baseline. According to the *Diagnostic and Statistical Manual of Mental Disorders, Fifth Edition, Text Revision* (*DSM-5-TR*), there must be 5 or more symptoms including depressed mood, weight loss/decreased appetite, fatigue, or feelings of worthlessness. Refer to the *DSM-5-TR* for the full criteria.[7]

A low mood can be a normal reaction to a challenging situation, including a new chronic medical diagnosis.[2–4] The symptoms reported here could be a sign of an adjustment disorder, which is characterized by emotional or behavioral symptoms developing in response to a stressor within 3 months of its onset and terminating by 6 months after the stressor's end. It typically evolves when coping with change is hard and temporarily interferes with psychosocial functioning. The distress experienced is out of proportion to the severity of the stressor and causes significant impairment.[5]

It can be typical for a patient to experience anxiety related to a new diagnosis, especially one that interferes with social functioning or is obvious to others because of the disease's physical presentation or its treatment. Anxiety related to a new diagnosis should not cause significant distress or functional impairment and should resolve in less than 6 months.[8] However, social anxiety disorder is characterized by a marked anxiety about social situations in which the individual is exposed to possible scrutiny by others and the individual fears they will act in a way or show anxiety symptoms that will be negatively evaluated.[9] Given that social situations almost always provoke this fear, these situations are avoided. The fear must be out of proportion to the actual threat posed by the situation, cause distress, and be persistent for at least 6 months.

For London, an adjustment disorder could be the right diagnostic fit, as she has experienced a new change with her NG tube, along with physical and behavioral changes over the past 2 months. However, it will be important to rule out depression or suicidal ideation given her more recent statement.

Screening London with the PHQ-A can provide clarity toward a depression diagnosis and the ASQ can potentially identify any concerns for suicidal ideation.[10] A helpful clinical pathway for the evaluation and treatment of patients at risk for depression can be found online (www.chop.edu/clinical-pathway/depression-clinical-pathway).

London's dad is wondering how a person can tell the difference between a "depressed mood" and a "normal moody tween."

While preadolescents and adolescents may show some mood lability, irritability, or melancholy, these symptoms should be intermittent and transient, unlike with MDD, when symptoms are present most of the day, nearly every day. While an adolescent may seem to have a low mood occasionally, they should demonstrate an improved mood when offered preferred or pleasurable activities. When in doubt, the caregiver can examine how the youth seems when with their peers, as this should be a time when they appear happy and engaged. Teachers or coaches may also be able to give insight into the adolescent's mood when caregivers are not around. Also, with patient permission, the clinician can consider sharing results of the screening measures with caregivers so families can better understand the concerns and diagnostic criteria as they relate to their child's symptoms.

Keep in Mind: Talking With Preadolescents and Adolescents

When talking with adolescents in a clinical interview, clinicians will often get a 1-word response, such as "OK," "Good," or "Fine." It is important to take the conversation further by having multiple ways to ask questions in a nonthreatening and creative manner. For example, when a clinician asks a teen about sleep, a common answer is "It's OK," but when the clinician probes further, they can usually find some aspects of sleep hygiene that could be improved (eg, using electronics until late hours, watching TV, difficulty initiating sleep). Some questions to ask include

- What time do you get into bed, and how long do you think it is until you fall asleep?
- Where do you do your homework?

Children and adolescents do not always identify as having a depressed mood.[10] They may describe a feeling of "blah" or "meh." The clinician can ask, "Tell me what feeling 'meh' means to you," as a way of getting more details. The depressed mood may be inferred through nonverbal communication such as facial expressions, body language, and sudden changes in appearance and demeanor. Some children and adolescents have irritability, which caregivers may describe as anger, blaming others, or getting easily frustrated over minor issues, but it should look different from typical frustration, as it is persistent and pervasive.[4]

Similarly, a markedly diminished interest or pleasure in activities may not be reported.[10] This may present as giving up on hobbies or quitting activities such as sports teams or withdrawing from social groups/clubs. A teen may say, "I used to play soccer," when the clinician asks if they play sports, and this is the clinician's opportunity to probe into why the teen no longer plays. Sleep changes can also be a clue to potential mood issues; both hypersomnia and hyposomnia are symptoms worth exploring.[4,7]

••• Communication Pearl ••• Social Media and Mood

It's crucial to understand the importance that social media plays in the lives of preadolescents and adolescents. Even if your patient is not active on social media, it's nearly impossible for youth to be completely removed from and unaffected by it. From bullying to body image comparison to gender and sexuality, it's important to ask young patients about their social media experiences and the potential connection to their mood and self-esteem. Social media use, especially early in adolescence, has been associated with higher depression, self-injurious thoughts, substance use, and poorer self-perception.[11]

In addition to discussing the risks of social media with patients, encourage the caregivers of your patients to take an active role in understanding their child's social media use and talk about how it is affecting their child's psychosocial functioning.

Back to the Case: Depression

You decide to screen London using the validated tools PHQ-A and ASQ to assess her depressive symptoms and possible suicidal ideation. She scores 13 (moderate depressive symptoms) on the PHQ-A and endorses recurrent thoughts of death over the past 2 weeks. London seems to meet criteria for MDD given her symptoms of low mood, anhedonia, weight loss, low energy, and recurrent thoughts of death for at least 2 weeks that are causing impairment and distress.[7] You make this assessment after scoring her results, the direct clinical interview with the London and her father, assessment of her functional impairment in different domains, and consideration for other psychiatric conditions.[10] (Refer to Chapter 5, Somatic Symptoms and Depression, for the assessment of functioning and impairment of depressive disorders.)

➤ How do you know that her symptoms are not related to her chronic illness and that she has a separate diagnosis of depression?

This is a very important question when working with patients who have chronic illness and mental health concerns and/or disorders, as depression and physical health issues can have a robust cyclical relationship. A physical issue can affect quality of life, leading to depressive symptoms, and the depressive symptoms can affect adherence to treatment and stamina to deal with chronic illness, potentially making it worse.[2,3] If it felt unclear whether this was a stand-alone MDD diagnosis, you can make the provisional diagnosis of an adjustment disorder until it becomes clearer in time. However, given the length of time and the marked change in London's psychosocial functioning (eg, anhedonia, cessation of social activities, mood changes), plus her thoughts of dying, MDD is an appropriate diagnosis. Consultation with a mental health specialist and colleagues is always appropriate if you are unsure.

➤ London has been writing sad poems and has made statements about dying. How do you determine if this behavior is an indicator of suicidal ideation?

It is important to take this disclosure seriously and sensitively. If a screening tool such as the ASQ has not already been completed by the patient, this is an appropriate time to use it plus have a private talk with the patient. Some questions that could be asked include

- Can you share with me about your poems that talk about dying?
- How long have you felt this way?
- What do you know about your disease and how/if it can affect your life in such a way as to cause death?

- Do you feel like you would do anything to act on those thoughts?
- Do you think you're going to die because of your illness?
- Does dealing with your illness make you feel sad enough to do something to harm yourself or even end your life?
- Are there times when you feel like you'd be better off dead? Is that a constant feeling, or does it occur only when you're thinking about your illness?
- Have you talked with anyone about these feelings?

Regardless of the foundation for sad poems, if London is experiencing active suicidal ideation, it is important to conduct a brief suicide safety assessment, create a safety plan, and help connect her with resources immediately.[10,12] Refer to the online resource from the AAP "Conducting a Brief Suicide Safety Assessment" (www.aap.org/en/patient-care/blueprint-for-youth-suicide-prevention/strategies-for-clinical-settings-for-youth-suicide-prevention/conducting-a-brief-suicide-safety-assessment). Refer also to Chapter 9, Suicidality and Eating Disorder, for more information on suicidality.

Management: Depression

After making a diagnosis of depression, the clinician will want to determine the severity, as this will guide the management and treatment decisions they recommend. For a description of depression severity, refer to Chapter 5, Somatic Symptoms and Depression.

Mild cases of depression can be followed by active monitoring in the pediatric primary care setting. During this active monitoring phase, clinicians should frequently check in with patients, weekly or biweekly for 6 to 8 weeks, to monitor symptoms and offer support.[12] These check-ins can happen by telephone, video visit, or in-person visits. During this period, the management goals should be discussed so that the patient and caregivers have an individualized plan to follow.

Active monitoring can include offering support for lifestyle modifications, which can be done before initiating psychotherapeutic or pharmacological treatment of depression. Recommendations for support provided during active monitoring include

- Promotion of healthy habits
  - Nutrition—3 healthy meals and 2 healthy snacks, with adequate water intake and reduced caffeine and sugary drinks
  - Sleep hygiene—healthy sleep habits; consistent bedtime and wake times every day of the week; reduced or ceased daytime napping; using the bed only for sleep; reduction of electronics before sleep
  - Activity—a daily goal of moving the body (eg, taking a short walk, going outside in the morning, playing with the dog)

- Participating in hobbies/leisure/faith activities: clubs, sports, instrument lessons, religious groups
- Connecting with peer support groups within the community
- Developing problem-solving strategies and skills[10,12]
- Patient and/or family education on depression and suicidality, including giving crisis numbers[10,12]
- Safety planning[10]

In addition, accommodations at school (eg, reduced workloads, extended time on tests and location accommodations, frequent breaks, organization support, meetings with the school counselor, safety/crisis plans, modified school days) may be necessary during a time when MDD is interfering with functioning. Educate caregivers about their child's rights under the Individuals with Disabilities Act. An Individualized Education Program (IEP) or a 504 plan can be implemented to secure school supports. Refer to Chapter 8, Attention-Deficit/Hyperactivity Disorder and Learning Difficulties, for more information on IEPs and 504 plans. A collaborative relationship with the school (eg, guidance counselor, psychologist, social worker, and/or teacher) can be helpful. The AAP offers useful online resources for clinicians and caregivers.

- For clinicians: "Supporting Students with Depression in School" (www.aap.org/en/patient-care/school-health/mental-health-in-schools/supporting-students-with-depression-in-school)
- For caregivers: "IEPs and 504 Plans: A Guide for Parents" (www.healthychildren.org/English/health-issues/conditions/developmental-disabilities/Pages/Individualized-Education-Program.aspx)

The clinician will also want to work closely with London's gastroenterologist to ensure that her IBD is being managed appropriately. Flares of IBD can be related to worsening of depression symptoms. Refer to Chapter 11, Depression and Depressive Disorder, for information on the treatment plan for depression, including psychotherapy and psychopharmacology.

For patients who have reached the threshold at which they would benefit from therapy, the recommendations are cognitive behavioral therapy, interpersonal psychotherapy for adolescents, or dialectical behavior therapy.[4,12]

Brief interventions: While the patient is awaiting an appointment with a mental health specialist, there are some brief interventions that can be introduced in the office setting to help improve functioning. These include

- **Behavioral activation**
  — The goal is to help your patient in identifying rewarding or enjoyable activities to help reduce their anhedonia/avoidance behaviors and subsequently devise strategies to enhance their motivation to complete them.

- Examples include going on a walk with a friend to get ice cream once this week, spending phone-free time with the family during dinnertime, or baking cookies—small goals that can be worked into a daily schedule.
- In addition to performing the activity, pairing it with a reflective exercise is recommended, such as journaling or creating a mood log to help keep track of how the activities affect their mood.

- **Problem-solving**
  - Help the patient identify a problem, then work with them to create strategies to help solve the problem.
  - For example, London discussed feeling like she cannot invite friends over due to her messy bedroom. It's possible to use problem-solving to help her address this issue (cleaning her room) while also addressing behavioral activation (eg, doing an activity that will feel rewarding when completed). This can help increase self-efficacy and boost coping skills. Problem-solving can be helpful for both small steps (cleaning room) and bigger ones (increasing social interactions).
- **Relaxation techniques**
  - Introduce deep breathing, meditation, or a grounding technique as a way to help calm the mind and body when feeling overwhelmed, sad, or hopeless.
    - *Deep breathing:* Teach the patient to breathe in slowly through their nose for the count of 5 ("smell the flower") and breathe out slowly through their mouth for the count of 5 ("blow off the petals").
    - *Grounding:* 5-4-3-2-1 method—Identify 5 things you see, 4 things you feel, 3 things you hear, 2 things you smell, and 1 thing you taste.

➤ How long is a major depressive episode likely to last?

The median duration of depression is between 4 and 8 months, with untreated episodes likely lasting longer.[7] Reassuringly, 90% of MDD episodes remit within 1 to 2 years, while only 6% to 10% become chronic.[4] The length of the episode can be affected by many factors, including health, symptom severity, treatment readiness and effectiveness, and psychosocial support.

Conclusion

In this case, a patient with a low mood in the setting of chronic illness was diagnosed with depression, after an adjustment disorder was considered as a possible diagnosis. The evolution of her mood symptoms highlights the need for repeated screenings over time, especially of youth at risk for depression because of chronic disease. Screening for suicidal ideation should always accompany depression screening, and having frequent check-ins to ask about depressive symptoms and suicidal thoughts is a helpful way to address these issues with adolescents. The mental health concerns of patients with chronic illness are best managed when primary care clinicians and specialists (medical and mental/behavioral health) work collaboratively.

Lessons Learned From the Rain Cloud

In the Rain Cloud case (as depression of chronic disease unfolds), depression interferes with the joy of a sunny day, causing low mood, loss of pleasure in activities, and a number of other symptoms that interfere with daily functioning, such as loss of appetite, poor sleep, and withdrawal from social activities. It is important to monitor for bigger storms, including self-harm and suicidality, while screening for common coexisting conditions, including anxiety. With behavioral activation strategies and appropriate treatment, the rainy days will pass.

- Chronic disease increases the risk for depression.[2–4]
- Mood lability may be common around puberty but should be intermittent, transient, and not interfering with peer interactions.
- Screening for anxiety, depression, and suicidality should occur simultaneously, as these commonly coexist.[10,12–14]
- Safety planning should be done for all patients with depression.[10,12–14]
- Brief interventions in the office may include behavioral activation, relaxation skills, and problem-solving to increase coping skills and self-efficacy.[10,12–14]

Keywords: adjustment disorder, chronic disease, chronic illness, depression, social anxiety disorder, suicidality

Suggested Reading

American Academy of Pediatrics. Suicide: Blueprint for Youth Suicide Prevention. Accessed April 6, 2026. https://www.aap.org/en/patient-care/blueprint-for-youth-suicide-prevention

Dudeney J, Aaron RV, Hathway T, et al. Anxiety and depression in youth with chronic pain: a systematic review and meta-analysis. *JAMA Pediatr*. 2024;178(11):1114–1123 PMID: 39250143

Perzow SED, Hu J, Bristol M, et al. Systematic review and meta-analysis of psychological interventions for depression symptoms in young people with long-term physical health conditions. *J Pediatr Psychol*. 2025;50(7):699–714 PMID: 40795045

Substance Abuse and Mental Health Services Administration. Behavioral health resources for youth: children and youth mental health. Updated April 17, 2024. Accessed April 6, 2026. https://www.samhsa.gov/mental-health/children-and-families/school-health/resources

Terman M, Terman JS, Quitkin FM, McGrath PJ, Stewart JW, Rafferty B. Light therapy for seasonal affective disorder: a review of efficacy. *Neuropsychopharmacology*. 1989;2(1):1–22 PMID: 2679625

Walter HJ, Abright AR, Bukstein OG, et al. Clinical practice guideline for the assessment and treatment of children and adolescents with major and persistent depressive disorders. *J Am Acad Child Adolesc Psychiatry*. 2023;62(5):479–502 PMID: 36273673

Xu T, Chen Y, Shen Q, Dai S, Yan H, Ren J. A systematic review and meta-analysis of anxiety and depression in children and adolescents with inflammatory bowel disease: prevalence and association. *J Psychiatr Res*. 2026;196:78–89 PMID: 41687568

References

1. Grillo TG, Almeida LR, Beraldo RF, et al. Heart failure as an adverse effect of infliximab for Crohn's disease: a case report and review of the literature. *World J Clin Cases*. 2021;9(33):10382–10391 PMID: 34904114
2. Benton T, Staab J, Evans DL. Medical co-morbidity in depressive disorders. *Ann Clin Psychiatry*. 2007;19(4):289–303 PMID: 18058286
3. National Institute of Mental Health. *Understanding the Link Between Chronic Disease and Depression*. National Institutes of Health; 2024. NIH publication 24-MH-8015. Accessed February 6, 2026. https://www.nimh.nih.gov/health/publications/chronic-illness-mental-health
4. Shatkin JP. Depression. In: *Child and Adolescent Health: A Practical All-in-One Guide*. WW Norton & Co; 2015:199–231
5. American Psychiatric Association. Adjustment disorders. In: *Diagnostic and Statistical Manual of Mental Disorders*. 5th ed, text rev. American Psychiatric Association Publishing; 2022:319
6. Van Hedger K, Mayo LM, Bershad AK, Madray R, de Wit H. Effects of acute drug administration on emotion: a review of pharmacological MRI studies. *Curr Addict Rep*. 2021;8(2):181–193 PMID: 34631363
7. American Psychiatric Association. Major depressive disorder. In: *Diagnostic and Statistical Manual of Mental Disorders*. 5th ed, text rev. American Psychiatric Association Publishing; 2022:183
8. American Psychiatric Association. Anxiety disorder due to another medical condition. In: *Diagnostic and Statistical Manual of Mental Disorders*. 5th ed, text rev. American Psychiatric Association Publishing; 2022:259
9. American Psychiatric Association. Social anxiety disorder. In: *Diagnostic and Statistical Manual of Mental Disorders*. 5th ed, text rev. American Psychiatric Association Publishing; 2022:229
10. Zuckerbrot RA, Cheung A, Jensen PS, Stein REK, Laraque D; GLAD-PC Steering Group. Guidelines for Adolescent Depression in Primary Care (GLAD-PC), I: practice preparation, identification, assessment, and initial management. *Pediatrics*. 2018;141(3):e20174081 PMID: 29483200
11. Teague S, Somoray K, Shatte A, et al. Digital media use and child health and development: a systematic review and meta-analysis. *JAMA Pediatr*. 2026;e260085 PMID: 41801211
12. Cheung AH, Zuckerbrot RA, Jensen PS, Laraque D, Stein REK; GLAD-PC Steering Group. Guidelines for Adolescent Depression in Primary Care (GLAD-PC), II: treatment and ongoing management. *Pediatrics*. 2018;141(3):e20174082 PMID: 29483201
13. Sun Y, Kong Z, Song Y, Liu J, Wang X. The validity and reliability of the PHQ-9 on screening of depression in neurology: a cross sectional study. *BMC Psychiatry*. 2022;22(1):98 PMID: 35139810
14. Foy JM, Green CM, Earls MF; American Academy of Pediatrics Committee on Psychosocial Aspects of Child and Family Health and Mental Health Leadership Work Group. Mental health competencies for pediatric practice. *Pediatrics*. 2019;144(5):e20192757 PMID: 31636143

CHAPTER 7

Irritable Mood

The Wind: Characterized by intense bursts of wind that can cause disruption to order or be hard to settle. Look out for disruptive behavior or irritability, followed by periods of calm.

Presentation

Kingston is a 2½-year-old whose grandmother brings him to see you because he throws excessive tantrums. His grandmother reports that she raised 3 children and one had outbursts similar to those of Kingston, but she never knew what caused these bursts of anger and aggression and wants to know if Kingston has a diagnosis of anything. Kingston is described as going from 0 to 100 quickly, and when he isn't getting his way, he will cry, hit, throw things, and bite people. He doesn't recover easily from these tantrums, and sometimes they will last for an hour. When Kingston is doing preferred activities, his mood is pleasant. He's very active. He loves to run, climb, and test limits at the playground, such as jumping off the apparatus. His grandmother feels that she always needs to watch him closely, so he doesn't get hurt or doesn't hurt other children.

Patient History and Review of Systems

- **Birth history:** full term, no complications
- **Medical history:** atopic dermatitis
- **Family history:** mother with attention-deficit/hyperactivity disorder (ADHD)
- **Social history:** lives at home with his 18-year-old mother and grandmother
- **Constitutional:** no fevers, weight loss/gain, or night sweats
- **HEENT:** no vision or hearing changes
- **Respiratory:** no cough or shortness of breath
- **Gastrointestinal:** no vomiting, constipation, or diarrhea
- **Integumentary:** eczematous patches on extremities
- **Lymphatic:** no enlarged lymph nodes
- **Neurological:** no headaches

Kingston was born at full term to a 16-year-old mother and is being raised by his mother and maternal grandmother. He has a history of atopic dermatitis but is otherwise healthy and takes no medications. He is growing well and has healthy nutrition and effective sleep hygiene.

➤ **What organic diseases may have behavioral manifestations, and how do these mimic or co-occur with behavioral or developmental disorders?**

Differential Diagnosis

This case focuses mostly on behavioral symptoms, including tantrums, with bursts of anger and aggression, and hyperactivity. While a behavioral diagnosis is likely, consider possible organic pathologies that may have behavioral manifestations, as well as developmental disorders.

- **Tantrums:** A developmentally appropriate response to handling big emotions without cognitive and language skills to manage these emotions. Typically start around 12 to 18 months of age, worsen between 2 and 3 years, and taper or resolve by 3½ years, as language skills improve. They could be a reaction to everyday parenting, such as limit setting and discipline, as well as broader issues such as family dynamics, family changes, and disruption in daily life or routines.

- **Atopic dermatitis flares:** Children with severe atopic dermatitis flares can feel intensely itchy and uncomfortable, which can lead to behavioral changes and/or sleep disturbances. As a toddler, this patient may not yet be able to articulate that his irritability is caused by skin irritation and fatigue.
- **Sleep issues:** Poor sleep hygiene and insufficient sleep, or sleep apnea, which can affect mood and behavior regulation.
- **Speech delay:** Delays in speech can affect behavior by increasing frustrations around communication difficulties.
- **Attention-deficit/hyperactivity disorder:** Persistent pattern of inattention and/or hyperactivity/impulsivity that interferes with functioning or development. Several symptoms present before age 12 years, in 2 or more settings, and interfere with or impair the quality of social, academic, or occupational functioning.[1]
- **Adjustment disorder:** The development of emotional or behavioral symptoms in response to an identifiable stressor within 3 months of the stressor's onset.[2]
- **Reactive attachment disorder:** Social disinhibition and lack of enduring relationships. In a toddler, this may look like minimally seeking or responding to comfort when distressed. May have periods of unexplained irritability.[3]
- **Disruptive mood dysregulation disorder (DMDD):** Characterized by severe, recurrent outbursts verbally or behaviorally that are out of proportion to the situation or provocation. These outbursts are inconsistent with the developmental level and occur 3 or more times per week on average. In between outbursts, the baseline mood is persistently irritable or angry most of the time. Impulsiveness and disorganized attention are not essential features.[4]
- **Oppositional defiant disorder (ODD):** Characterized by resisting or conforming to others' demands. Often loses temper, blames others for mistakes, and argues with adults. Mood can often be described as easily annoyed, angry, resentful, or spiteful.[5]
- **Posttraumatic stress disorder:** Concentration difficulties, restlessness, irritability, and inattention may be present.[6]
- **Autism spectrum disorder (ASD):** May demonstrate inattention, impaired social relationships, communication difficulties, and difficult behaviors.[2] May have tantrums caused by inability to tolerate change.[7]
- **Trauma:** Past traumatic experiences can affect the child's feeling of safety and present with disruptive or irritable behavior.
- **Anxiety:** Disruptive behaviors or irritable mood can be a reaction to being faced with demands that make someone anxious. Anxiety can also present with inattention.

- **New-onset chronic illness or pain:** Diseases that cause persistent discomfort or pain may cause an irritable mood, restlessness, or inattention.
- **Seizure/epilepsy:** Seizures can cause lapses in awareness that look like inattention. Epilepsy also occurs at elevated rates in children with ADHD.[1]
- **Medication-induced symptoms:** Medications such as bronchodilators, isoniazid, antipsychotics, and thyroid replacement can cause symptoms of inattention, hyperactivity, or impulsivity that can mimic ADHD symptoms.[1]

Kingston's grandmother recalls that his mother had similar behaviors when she was young and wonders if he could have ADHD.

➤ **Should Kingston be evaluated for ADHD?**

Evaluation

Kingston's age is a critical piece of the clinician's evaluation and diagnostic decision-making because some of his behaviors are age appropriate. Attention-deficit/hyperactivity disorder begins in childhood and cannot be diagnosed if there is an absence of any symptoms before 12 years.[1] In most cases, it is not diagnosed until around age 6 years, while in kindergarten, but can be diagnosed beginning around age 4 or 5 years depending on symptom history and impairment level.[1,8] Key elements to consider in the history eliciting and observation include

- What are his behaviors like in different settings? Is the behavior the same at home, in child care, and with other caregivers?
- How long have these behaviors occurred? Are they new or a response to a change, such as a new living situation or change in home structure?
- What are the triggers or antecedents of his behaviors? Does the behavior always happen when he is tired or hungry, or are there other identifiable patterns?
- How do his caregivers respond to these behaviors? Is aggression met with aggression? Have behavior management strategies been implemented?
- Are there potential medical causes of his behavioral concerns? Ask about signs and symptoms of sleep apnea, nutritional deficiencies, hearing or vision concerns, and/or chronic pain. Does he have a medical diagnosis such as asthma or diabetes that is untreated or is chronic and continues to be symptomatic despite treatment?
- Has he had any exposure to trauma or adverse childhood experiences? For example, has he witnessed or experienced abuse or violence?

Back to the Case: Age-Appropriate Behaviors

Kingston may be too young to receive a diagnosis of ADHD, and with his baseline mood being happy, he does not meet criteria for DMDD.[4] It seems there is not a *Diagnostic and Statistical Manual of Mental Disorders, Fifth Edition, Text Revision* (*DSM-5-TR*) diagnosis for his behaviors yet, but you can explain to his grandmother that you will continue to monitor his symptoms and see how they evolve as he ages. Attention-deficit/hyperactivity disorder is most often diagnosed during elementary school when children struggle with attention and behavior in the classroom and at home and these behaviors significantly interfere with functioning in these or other settings. Additionally, given the family history of ADHD, it will be important to keep this diagnosis in mind as he matures.

➤ **What strategies can you offer Kingston's grandmother to help manage his behavior at this age?**

Management: Age-Appropriate Behaviors

Providing Kingston's grandmother with behavior management strategies can help her set realistic expectations to manage his tantrums. Here are some examples of ways to help caregivers navigate strong emotions and tantrums.

- First and foremost, it's important to **stay calm.** When children are young and feeling out of control, it can be helpful to remember that their brain is still developing, particularly their prefrontal cortex, which helps with planning, organization, and regulation. A tantrum is like a giant windstorm of feelings, created by a child's underdeveloped nervous system, and they are wrapped up in a vortex of overwhelming and wind-whipping emotion. The only way past it is through it. And if you can lend them your calm nervous system in that moment, it will help decrease intense negative emotional reactions and model positive emotion regulation skills. You can even narrate what you are doing to stay calm, such as "I'm going to take a deep breath and count to 10" or "I'm going to sit here and take deep breaths until you're ready for a hug."
- Try not to demand answers; **validate emotions.** Asking "Why are you upset?" in the middle of a tantrum is like shouting into the wind. There will be a time to ask questions, but not in the moment. Validate that the child is feeling strong emotions, such as "You look really angry" or "It's OK to cry when you feel sad." Remember, all feelings are OK, but all behaviors are not. Validating the emotion can help slow down the tantrum.

- **Redirection/distraction** can be a powerful technique to help a child move through a tantrum. Something such as "Let's set a timer for angry time, then we can do something else. Can you get me the timer?" or "Look at this new super-silly face I just learned to make" may work. Be creative; this can really help the child snap out of it.
- Be ready for **hugs.** Tantrums can feel overwhelming, so when the child is calmer, sometimes they just need a deep hug or another form of comfort from someone they trust. Get down to their level and remind them that they are loved and that it's going to be OK.
- **Delayed meaning making:** Find another time to identify the trigger. Not all tantrums have a "why" and "what's next," and that's OK. At age 2½ years, the importance of why can be addressed in a simple manner when the child is calm and the what's next can be kept very short. For example, if Kingston says he was angry because he did not get to open the door first, his grandmother can say, "Thank you for telling me that opening the door first was important to you. Next time, we will try to remember that, so you can go first."
- Kingston may benefit from supportive therapies such as occupational therapy, play therapy, and/or speech therapy—all of which can help improve overall developmental functioning.

Back to the Case: Potential ADHD

Kingston is now 6 years old and in first grade. After your discussion when he was a toddler, his grandmother and mother sought behavioral support from a therapist. They learned how to help him navigate his tantrums, how to help him increase his communication skills, and how to provide appropriate behavioral support such as special playtime, with lots of opportunity for physical activity. He even participated in a social skills group and has made some meaningful friendships with peers. He has continued to be an active child, and although he has had episodes of outbursts, his grandmother and mother feel better equipped to manage them. However, his first grade teacher is concerned that Kingston is getting into trouble more than his peers. According to the teacher, Kingston needs reminders to pay attention and to remain in his seat. The family has received a few phone calls about Kingston getting angry in school and pushing peers or taking toys. Last week, he threw a rock on the playground, and it hit another child; and today, his grandmother got a phone call that he knocked over other kids' block tower during free play. Kingston says he doesn't know why he does these things, and he says he wants to be a good boy. Kingston's teacher wants to know where these newer aggressive and disruptive behaviors are coming from when he knows the school rules.

Discussion: Potential ADHD

Children with ADHD have trouble with impulse control.[2,8,9] In this case, Kingston likely had trouble holding himself back or taking a moment to think about the rules. He understands the rules but lacks the executive function skills to resist an impulse and consider the consequences of following this impulse.

Keep in Mind: Stigmatization of Children With ADHD

Children with ADHD can be stigmatized as "bad" or "problem" children. They may get into trouble more than peers and may therefore get a negative reputation at school and with friends' caregivers. It is important to distinguish the behavior from the person. It is helpful to praise children who have ADHD for their strengths and when they are controlling their impulses, so they hear positive aspects of themselves from caregivers and authority figures, to maintain a positive self-esteem and self-worth.[2,8–10]

Management of this behavior should be focused on helping build executive function skills, rather than reciting the rules. Games such as freeze dance, red light/green light, Simon says, board games (eg, word games, chess), and puzzles can help children build these types of skills by working on planning, organization, problem-solving, sustained attention, and turn taking—all of which are crucial to executive function skill development.

Kingston's mother and grandmother are concerned that he has autism because he has trouble making friends, prefers to be alone, and is extremely hyperfocused on activities. For example, they report that he would rather build with a block set for 2 hours than go to the playground with other kids. They would like to know if this is a sign of autism.

Children with ADHD and ASD can be hyperfocused on preferred tasks. Unlike with children on the autism spectrum, though, the activities that children with ADHD concentrate on are age and developmentally appropriate.[8,11] For example, a 6-year-old with ADHD may have a deep interest in a fictional character (eg, Harry Potter) or a certain video game, while a 6-year-old on the spectrum may be highly focused on train schedules (eg, being able to identify many types of trains, the routes they take, and the corresponding times for each route), which is different for a child their age. Additionally, the play of children with ADHD is typically functionable (eg, learning how mechanisms work by opening and closing a door) and not exploratory (eg, spinning a wheel and staring closely at it) like the play of children with ASD is.

Impaired social communication is a key diagnostic feature of ASD and may cause difficulty making or keeping friends.[7] In contrast, children with ADHD may have difficulty making or keeping friends because of their behavior impulsivity or frequent interruption of others in conversation.[8,11]

Further, while children on the autism spectrum may be focused on a particular topic, children with ADHD can easily talk about many topics and have a back-and-forth conversation.[1,8]

➤ What additional evaluation can you do to determine a diagnosis for Kingston?

Refer to the Appendix for links to the following tools online:

- **NICHQ Vanderbilt Assessment Scale:** Screening questionnaire to diagnose and monitor ongoing ADHD symptoms, including hyperactivity, impulsivity, and inattention; parent and teacher versions; for use in children 6 to 12 years of age.
- **Social Communication Questionnaire (SCQ):** Screening tool to evaluate communication skills and social functioning in children 4 years and older who may have ASD; designed to be administered by psychologists, psychiatrists, or special education teachers; 40 questions, typically completed by the parent.
- **Strengths and Difficulties Questionnaire (SDQ):** A general behavioral screening questionnaire, for children and adolescents aged 2 to 17 years, that focuses on emotional symptoms, conduct, hyperactivity/impulsivity, peer relationships, and prosocial behavioral concerns.
  — 25 items; can be completed by parents, teachers, or child (age dependent)

Back to the Case: ADHD

At your suggestion, Kingston's mom and teacher each completed the NICHQ Vanderbilt Assessment Scale. The results are shown in Table 7-1. His mom and teacher scored him high for inattentive and hyperactive/impulsive symptoms, which suggests he has ADHD, combined subtype.

Table 7-1. Kingston's Scores on the NICHQ Vanderbilt Assessment Scale

Items	Parent	Teacher
Scored 2 or 3 for questions 1–9 (inattentive symptoms)	6	7
Scored 2 or 3 for questions 10–18 (hyperactive/impulsive symptoms)	9	6
Scored 4 or 5 for questions 48–55 (impairment scores)	4	5

Abbreviation: NICHQ, National Institute for Children's Health Quality.

Attention-deficit/hyperactivity disorder is diagnosed by a persistent pattern of inattention and hyperactivity/impulsivity that occurs in 2 or more settings (typically home and school).[1] On the rating scale, it is important to understand how it is scored. For the 9 items related to inattention and the 9 related to hyperactivity/impulsivity, the questionnaire looks at meeting symptom thresholds (eg, ≥6 rated at a numerical value of 2 ["often"] or 3 ["very often"]) and not total scale score or cutoff.

Symptoms of inattention may include

- Mistakes on typically automatic tasks or inattention to detail on assignments
- Not following directions
- Difficulty with organization
- Easily distracted

Symptoms of hyperactivity/impulsivity may include

- Fidgeting
- Difficulty staying seated
- Always on the go
- Blurting out answers
- Trouble taking turns

Additionally, symptoms need to interfere with daily functioning and be present for at least 6 months, beginning before age 12 years.[1] The symptoms should not be exclusively due to another psychiatric or medical disorder. Based on these results and your clinical assessment, Kingston meets criteria for ADHD, combined subtype.[1,8] Refer to the *DSM-5-TR* for full diagnostic criteria.

➤ **How should a clinician respond when a caregiver asks if they "caused" their child's ADHD?**

Discussion: ADHD

First, reassure the caregiver that they did not cause the ADHD. Even when risk factors are present, that does not mean that all children with those risk factors will be diagnosed with ADHD. Then, explain that ADHD is considered a neurodevelopmental disorder, which essentially means that there are some environmental, genetic, and physiological risk factors for ADHD and that the symptoms may change over time.[1,8]

- **Environmental:** Very low birth weight, preterm birth, prenatal exposure to smoking, neurotoxin exposure (eg, lead), infection (eg, encephalitis), in utero alcohol exposure.
- **Genetic:** Heritability of ADHD is approximately 74%, according to the *DSM-5-TR*. There is no single gene responsible for ADHD.
- **Physiological:** Some conditions may influence or elevate ADHD symptoms, including being blind or deaf/hard of hearing, metabolic abnormalities, nutritional deficiencies, and epilepsy.

Management: ADHD

Current American Academy of Pediatrics guidelines recommend behavior therapy that focuses on parent training as the first line of treatment for children with ADHD 6 years and younger, before medication is started. For children older than 6 years, the recommendation includes behavior therapy and medication, plus collaboration with schools.[8] (Refer to Chapter 12, Attention-Deficit/Hyperactivity Disorder, for more information on managing ADHD.)

- Psychosocial interventions
  - Behavior therapy such as Behavioral Parent Training/Parent Management Training (BPT/PMT), Parent-Child Interaction Therapy (PCIT), and the Positive Parenting Program (Triple P)
  - School/classroom accommodations, such as a 504 plan, Individualized Education Program, and/or school-based counseling
  - Social skills groups
  - Occupational therapy
- Medication options
  - Stimulant medications
  - Non-stimulant medications

Back to the Case: Worsening Symptoms or a Coexisting Condition

Kingston is now 8 years old. Over the past 2 years, he made significant strides in his academic performance. Last year, his grandmother and mother worked with the school to implement a 504 plan with accommodations such as extended time on tests, preferential seating, and distraction-free testing environments. In addition, he met with the school counselor monthly for a social skills "lunch bunch" group, which helped improved his relationship with his peers and increased his frustration tolerance. Outside of school, Kingston and his caregivers completed a course of BPT, which helped them learn to manage his irritability and executive functioning challenges. He was also enrolled in a karate class and worked hard on achieving his belts. Last year, he started taking methylphenidate and his caregivers and teachers agree that the methylphenidate works well on school days, and they give him medication "holidays" when he's not in school.

Despite all this progress, his caregivers are now concerned about his mood. When younger, he was always described as a "happy kid," but now it seems as if his baseline mood is grumpy and argumentative. He seems to hate it when his schedule is changed, and he becomes angry. His caregivers say they have become so tired of fighting with him that they often give in and let him play video games all day rather than argue about doing non-preferred tasks.

Keep in Mind: The Anger Iceberg

Anger is a basic emotion felt by everyone but may be the outward manifestation of many other emotions that are under the surface. This is known as the Anger Iceberg.[12] Caregivers can think of the anger they see as an expression of the raw feelings underneath. It can be helpful for them to try to name emotions other than anger that a child may be experiencing, such as sadness, frustration, or embarrassment, to help the child connect to these emotions rather than display anger. Further, when caregivers can identify the underlying emotions, they are often better able to also identify triggers and minimize obstacles.

➤ **Is ADHD likely to be causing his angry outbursts or could there be another coexisting condition?**

Additional Differential Diagnosis: Worsening Symptoms or a Coexisting Condition

- **Worsening symptoms of ADHD**
- **Sleep disturbances/disorders**
- **Disruptive mood dysregulation disorder**
- **Anxiety**
- **Depression**
- **Oppositional defiant disorder**
- **Adjustment issues, such as changes in home environment, parenting styles, or home structure or daily routines**
- **Trauma exposure**
- **Peer issues/peer pressure**
- **Screen time and social media use**

Coexisting conditions are more common in girls with ADHD but occur frequently in both boys and girls.[1] Oppositional defiant disorder and ADHD co-occur in 50% of children with combined subtype and 25% of those with inattentive subtype, according to the *DSM-5-TR*.[1] While most children with DMDD have ADHD symptoms, fewer children with ADHD have DMDD symptoms.[1] Anxiety and depression are slightly more common in patients with ADHD than the general population.[1] In adolescents, substance use disorders are relatively more frequent than in the general population.[1] Other coexisting conditions to consider include epilepsy, sleep disorders, learning disorders, tic disorders, ASD, language disorders, and allergy/autoimmune disorders.[1]

Additional Evaluation: Worsening Symptoms or a Coexisting Condition

To further refine whether Kingston has worsening symptoms of ADHD or a coexisting condition as the explanation for his mood concerns and inflexibility, consider readministering the NICHQ Vanderbilt Assessment Scale to track his ADHD symptoms, or use one of the following screening tools to determine if he has symptoms of depression or anxiety. Refer to the Appendix for links to the tools online.

- **Pediatric Symptom Checklist-17 (PSC-17):** Widely used parent-completed measure of a child's psychosocial functioning, normed for children and adolescents aged 4 to 17 years, including internalized problems (eg, anxiety, depression), attention issues, and externalizing problems (eg, disruptive and oppositional behaviors). This is a briefer version of the PSC-35. Refer to Chapter 5, Somatic Symptoms and Depression, for additional details.
  - A score of 15 or higher suggests the need for further follow-up and an evaluation for the presence of a mental health disorder. Similarly, each subscale has a cutoff score.
    - Attention—7
    - Externalizing—7
    - Internalizing—5
- **Screen for Child Anxiety and Related Emotional Disorders (SCARED):** A pediatric anxiety screener used for children 8 years and older. A total score of 25 or higher may indicate the presence of an anxiety disorder. Child and parent rating scale versions are available.
  - Additionally, this screener will give the clinician subscale scores that may indicate a specific type of anxiety disorder such as generalized anxiety disorder, social anxiety disorder, panic, school anxiety, and separation anxiety.

If the additional screenings and evaluation do not raise a concern for another diagnosis, such as anxiety, depression, learning disability, or ODD, consider if a medication adjustment is warranted. This may involve increasing Kingston's current dosage or changing medication classes. For more on the medication management of ADHD, refer to Chapter 12, Attention-Deficit/Hyperactivity Disorder.

Conclusion

Attention-deficit/hyperactivity disorder symptoms may evolve and change throughout a person's lifespan, but what remains consistent is that there is impairment in more than one setting. In many cases, as with Kingston, clinicians can recognize that the ADHD symptoms presented during the toddler period, although the child was too young for that diagnosis. Psychosocial interventions, such as BPT or PCIT, can help caregivers manage their child's symptoms at these early ages, and then, as the child grows, interventions will include the participation of the child. While medication can be a treatment component, it is important to be well-versed in behavior management strategies, particularly for younger children.

Lessons Learned From the Wind

In the Wind case (as irritable mood unfolds), the mood can be wild and come in seemingly unpredictable bursts, but when caregivers are vigilant and study it, they can start to see patterns and teach themselves the best way to respond. In preparing to face the wind, they can keep the environment safe and comfortable for all.

- Tantrums are developmentally appropriate until age 3½ years, and when they persist beyond that, other diagnoses should be explored.
- Attention-deficit/hyperactivity disorder is characterized by inattention, hyperactivity, or both, occurring in more than one setting and impairing functioning in social, academic, and/or occupational settings.[1]
- Attention-deficit/hyperactivity disorder can coexist with many neurodevelopmental disorders, mental health diagnoses, and allergy/autoimmune conditions.[1,8]
- Given that ADHD symptoms can change across the developmental lifespan, iterative assessments are important to distinguish changing ADHD symptoms from coexisting diagnoses, as management will vary depending on the symptom cause.[1,8]
- Caregiver and teacher education on how to manage ADHD symptoms is crucial for success in managing symptoms, preserving self-esteem, and optimizing functioning across settings.[8,9]

Keywords: ADHD, DMDD, irritability, tantrums, Vanderbilt scales

Suggested Reading

American Academy of Pediatrics. Top tips for surviving tantrums. HealthyChildren.org. Updated April 21, 2021. Accessed April 7, 2026. https://www.healthychildren.org/English/family-life/family-dynamics/communication-discipline/Pages/Temper-Tantrums.aspx

Children and Adults with Attention-Deficit/Hyperactivity Disorder. 12 behavioral programs for managing ADHD. *ADHD Weekly*. June 29, 2017. Accessed February 9, 2026. https://chadd.org/adhd-weekly/12-behavioral-programs-for-managing-adhd

Lockwood K. Children's Hospital of Philadelphia. *Primary Care Perspectives*. ADHD medication management. June 13, 2023. Accessed February 9, 2026. https://www.podbean.com/media/share/pb-ssbjk-1544c61

Martin J, Langley K, Cooper M, et al. Sex differences in attention-deficit hyperactivity disorder diagnosis and clinical care: a national study of population healthcare records in Wales. *J Child Psychol Psychiatry*. 2024;65(12):1648–1658 PMID: 38864317

National Center for Health Statistics. Attention deficit hyperactivity disorder (ADHD). FastStats. Reviewed January 12, 2026. Accessed February 9, 2026. https://www.cdc.gov/nchs/fastats/adhd.htm

Power T, Wallace W, Volkert M, et al. Primary care clinical pathway for evaluation and treatment of attention-deficit/hyperactivity disorder (ADHD). Children's Hospital of Philadelphia. December 2024. Updated June 2025. Accessed February 9, 2026. https://www.chop.edu/clinical-pathway/adhd-clinical-pathway

Table 7. *DSM-IV* to *DSM-5* attention-deficit/hyperactivity disorder comparison. In: Ringeisen H, Casanueva C, Stambaugh L, Bose J, Hedden S; Center for Behavioral Health Statistics and Quality. DSM-5 *Changes: Implications for Child Serious Emotional Disturbance*. Substance Abuse and Mental Health Services Administration; 2016:17–20. Accessed February 9, 2026. https://www.ncbi.nlm.nih.gov/books/NBK519712/table/ch3.t3

References

1. American Psychiatric Association. Attention-deficit/hyperactivity disorder. In: *Diagnostic and Statistical Manual of Mental Disorders*. 5th ed, text rev. American Psychiatric Association Publishing; 2022:69–76
2. American Psychiatric Association. Adjustment disorders. In: *Diagnostic and Statistical Manual of Mental Disorders*. 5th ed, text rev. American Psychiatric Association Publishing; 2022:320–323
3. American Psychiatric Association. Reactive attachment disorder. In: *Diagnostic and Statistical Manual of Mental Disorders*. 5th ed, text rev. American Psychiatric Association Publishing; 2022:296–299
4. American Psychiatric Association. Disruptive mood dysregulation disorder. In: *Diagnostic and Statistical Manual of Mental Disorders*. 5th ed, text rev. American Psychiatric Association Publishing; 2022:179–183
5. American Psychiatric Association. Oppositional defiant disorder. In: *Diagnostic and Statistical Manual of Mental Disorders*. 5th ed, text rev. American Psychiatric Association Publishing; 2022:523–527
6. American Psychiatric Association. Posttraumatic stress disorder. In: *Diagnostic and Statistical Manual of Mental Disorders*. 5th ed, text rev. American Psychiatric Association Publishing; 2022:302–314

7. American Psychiatric Association. Autism spectrum disorder. In: *Diagnostic and Statistical Manual of Mental Disorders*. 5th ed, text rev. American Psychiatric Association Publishing; 2022:57–68
8. Wolraich ML, Hagan JF Jr, Allan C, et al; American Academy of Pediatrics Subcommittee on Children and Adolescents With Attention-Deficit/Hyperactivity Disorder. Clinical practice guideline for the diagnosis, evaluation, and treatment of attention-deficit/hyperactivity disorder in children and adolescents. *Pediatrics*. 2019;144(4):e20192528 PMID: 31570648
9. Centers for Disease Control and Prevention. Treatment of ADHD. Attention-Deficit/Hyperactivity Disorder (ADHD). May 16, 2024. Accessed February 9, 2026. https://www.cdc.gov/adhd/treatment/index.html
10. Wissow LS. Disruptive behavior and aggression. In: Foy JM, ed. *Mental Health Care of Children and Adolescents: A Guide for Primary Care Clinicians*. American Academy of Pediatrics; 2018:457–475
11. Power TJ, Mautone JA, Soffer SL. *Family-School Success for Children With ADHD: A Guide for Intervention*. Guilford Press; 2024
12. Benson K. The Anger Iceberg. The Gottman Institute. November 8, 2016. Updated January 16, 2026. Accessed February 9, 2026. https://www.gottman.com/blog/the-anger-iceberg

CHAPTER 8

Attention-Deficit/ Hyperactivity Disorder and Learning Difficulties

The Tornado: Characterized by chaotic, relentless energy. Look out for possible irritability with frustration especially around school and schoolwork.

Presentation

Denver is a 7-year-old second grader who is struggling in school. His teacher thinks that he isn't paying attention to her directions and then gets lost on the assignment. His class size is large, and the teacher reports that she does not always have time to repeat directions for him. At home, his parents struggle with getting him to follow household routines. For example, he often forgets to put on socks before coming downstairs for breakfast, or at night, he's told to brush his teeth and put on pajamas, but his parents will find him playing in the bathroom and forgetting what he was supposed to do. Denver's teacher reports that she once had a student with absence seizures who had similar behaviors of zoning out and missing directions, so she advised Denver's parents to bring him to the pediatrician.

Patient History and Review of Systems

- **Birth history:** 34-weeks'–gestation birth, 2,320-g birth weight, some apnea and bradycardia episodes in the neonatal intensive care unit (NICU), normal findings on head ultrasound, hyperbilirubinemia status post-phototherapy. No respiratory support needed. Spent 11 days in the NICU.
- **Medical history:** Developmental delays while receiving occupational therapy and speech therapy until age 2 years; now continues to receive only occupational therapy.
- **Social history:** Lives at home with his mom, dad, sister, and pet cat. No exposure to smoking, guns, or violence.
- **Medications:** None.

In addition, he has normal growth curves, with weight in the 35th percentile and height in the 75th percentile consistently, and his physical examination findings are normal.

➤ **What are common causes of significant school difficulties in a young child?**

Differential Diagnosis

- **Absence seizures:** Characterized by a brief seizure that looks similar to a sudden lapse in awareness, often with a blank stare and unresponsiveness. Can be mistaken for daydreaming. Afterward, the child has no memory of what happened during the event.
- **Hearing loss:** Denver is at risk because of his preterm birth and time in the NICU; can be seen in children with speech delay as well.
- **Neurodevelopmental disorder:** Denver's preterm birth and time in the NICU put him at risk for developmental delays. Prenatal drug or alcohol exposure is also a risk factor for a neurodevelopmental disorder, but there is no history of that given in this case. Repetitive motor behaviors, as seen in stereotypic movement disorder, Tourette syndrome, or autism spectrum disorder, should be distinguished from the fidgetiness of ADHD. Children with neurodevelopmental disorders can have impairment in social, occupational, and other areas of functioning without meeting all criteria for attention-deficit/hyperactivity disorder or a specific learning disorder.[1]

- **Oppositional defiant disorder (ODD):** Characterized by resisting conforming to others' demands. Children with this disorder often lose their temper, blame others for mistakes, and argue with adults.[2] It's important to understand the distinction between age-appropriate defiance and ODD, as this disorder is often misunderstood and overdiagnosed to describe nonspecific behavior problems that can be seen as on a spectrum and a "catchall" for difficult behaviors.[3] In this case, Denver's lack of following directions could be caused by resisting following the rules or directions of the adults in his life. He does not seem to have issues with his temper, though.
- **Attention-deficit/hyperactivity disorder (ADHD):** Persistent pattern of inattention and/or hyperactivity/impulsivity that interferes with functioning or development. Several symptoms present before age 12 years, in 2 or more settings, and interfere with or impair the quality of social, academic, or occupational functioning.[4] In this case, Denver is demonstrating symptoms of inattention but not hyperactivity or impulsivity, and these symptoms are impairing him at home and school.
- **Specific learning disorder (SLD):** A broad range of learning challenges that impede a child's ability to perform at the expected grade level or in concordance with their IQ. Preterm birth is a risk factor for learning disability.[5,6]
- **Anxiety disorder:** Children who struggle with attention, executive function, and learning can often feel anxious at school. It's important to learn if anxiety is contributing to the overall presentation or if there is a potential co-occurring anxiety disorder.[7]
- **Sleep disorder:** Sleep problems can contribute to inattention and poor school performance.
- **Delirium:** A disturbance in attention accompanied by reduced awareness of the environment, having developed over a short period and representing a change from baseline. Tends to fluctuate in severity throughout the day. Delirium is a direct physiological consequence of another condition, toxin, and/or substance, which, in this case, lacks evidence of being present.[8]
- **Trauma/posttraumatic stress:** Exposure to trauma or chronic stress can impact attention, executive functioning, and behavior regulation, which can affect learning and/or exacerbate learning challenges or disabilities. Additionally, early medical stress (eg, NICU hospitalization, maternal stress) and developmental vulnerability may increase risk. Trauma-related symptoms may occur even in the absence of known abuse or violence and warrant screening as a part of a comprehensive evaluation.[9,10]
- **Elevated blood lead concentration:** Elevated blood lead levels can lead to inattention, hyperactivity, impulsivity, and/or aggression. Even blood lead levels as low 1.3 mcg/dL (> 13 ppb) and up have been associated with behavioral symptoms, and approximately 1 in 5 cases of ADHD in the United States has been attributed to lead exposure.[11]

- **New-onset chronic illness or pain:** Diseases that cause persistent discomfort or pain may cause an irritable mood, restlessness, or inattention.
- **Hyperthyroidism:** Can cause inattention, restlessness, and sleep disturbance that can mimic ADHD symptoms. Other symptoms that do not fit with ADHD and that are not seen in this case include unexplained weight loss, heat intolerance, tremors, goiter, diarrhea, or proptosis.
- **Medication-induced symptoms:** Medications such as bronchodilators, isoniazid, antipsychotics, and thyroid replacement can cause symptoms of inattention, hyperactivity, or impulsivity that can mimic ADHD symptoms.[4]

➤ **Does Denver need further testing to narrow down the diagnosis?**

Evaluation

- **Absence seizures:** Denver's inattention does not seem consistent with absence seizures because he is not fully unresponsive during his periods of inattention. He can be seen doing other things while the teacher is giving instructions, and although he sometimes daydreams, calling his name will get him to respond. Therefore, an electroencephalogram is likely unnecessary.
- **Sleep disorder:** Denver's sleep hygiene should be explored further, as poor sleep can cause inattention and school difficulties. However, further eliciting of history determines that Denver is sleeping well. While he has a little trouble settling down to sleep, he typically sleeps 10 hours and sleeps through the night without waking. Therefore, a sleep study is likely unnecessary.
- **Hearing loss:** Findings from Denver's audiometric screenings at his primary care visits have all been normal. He does not have any speech difficulties and was cleared from speech therapy at age 2 years. Further audiological evaluation can be done, but it is unnecessary at this time.
- **Social history:** There is no history of trauma and the family did not endorse any additional familial or environmental stressors that may be contributing to his attention issues.
- **Elevated blood lead level:** Pediatric clinicians should do targeted screening for lead in individuals at high risk, which includes those with a developmental delay.[11]
- **Hyperthyroidism:** Thyroid function testing can be done based on clinical suspicion. Given that Denver does not have symptoms of hyperthyroidism beyond the behavioral symptoms, and has no family history of autoimmune disease, this testing is not necessary.

- **Attention-deficit/hyperactivity disorder:** Denver's behaviors are the same at home and school. His parents report that his inattention is not new and that he has always struggled with focusing. His symptoms seem consistent with ADHD. Further assessment is warranted; a parent and teacher should each complete the NICHQ Vanderbilt Assessment Scale (Table 8-1). Refer to the Appendix for a link to the tool online.
  - **NICHQ Vanderbilt Assessment Scale:** Screening questionnaire to diagnose and monitor ongoing ADHD symptoms, including hyperactivity, impulsivity, and inattention; parent and teacher versions; for use in children 6 to 12 years of age.

Table 8–1. Denver's Scores on the NICHQ Vanderbilt Assessment Scale

Item	Parent	Teacher
Scored 2 or 3 for questions 1–9 (inattentive symptoms)	7	8
Scored 2 or 3 for questions 10–18 (hyperactive/impulsive symptoms)	3	4
Scored 4 or 5 for questions 48–55 (impairment scores)	4	6

Abbreviation: NICHQ, National Institute for Children's Health Quality.

Denver's history, clinical assessment, and Vanderbilt scores are consistent with a diagnosis of ADHD, inattentive subtype. This subtype requires 6 or more of the inattentive symptoms to be present (eg, ≥6 items scored at a 2 or 3 across the 9 items) for at least 6 months to a degree that is inconsistent with developmental level and negatively affecting social and academic/occupational activities, plus significant impairment.[4,12] Refer to Chapter 7, Irritable Mood, for further diagnostic information for early assessment and diagnosis of ADHD, and Chapter 12, Attention-Deficit/Hyperactivity Disorder.

Keep in Mind: Coexisting Conditions

A diagnosis of ADHD can coexist with other neurodevelopmental conditions such as autism, sleep disorders, and/or medical conditions such as epilepsy. Attention-deficit/hyperactivity disorder also highly co-occurs with learning disabilities such as dyslexia, dyspraxia, and dyscalculia.[4,6]

Back to the Case: ADHD

Denver's parents have heard about ADHD and are worried about labeling him with this diagnosis because they feel that he will be treated differently at school. What psychoeducation can you provide them?

Discussion: ADHD

Being open about an ADHD diagnosis with Denver and his school helps reduce stigmatization and ensure accurate intervention. Although his parents are concerned that he will be treated differently, his teacher is already responding to him differently—and in a negative way—because of the classroom disruptions caused by his ADHD symptoms. It can help to provide parents with an example so they better understand this point, such as likening his ADHD diagnosis to a patient newly diagnosed with diabetes. If Denver had diabetes and was insulin dependent, most families would not hesitate to provide the school this information, as it affects his health and overall performance in school, so similarly, his school should know about his ADHD diagnosis. Denver should also be told about his diagnosis because not understanding his ADHD diagnosis, especially because it is a mental health diagnosis, may affect his own sense of self-efficacy, as he is receiving negative feedback and noticing that tasks may be harder for him than his peers. Giving him a diagnosis will help him get the support and services he needs to succeed in school and at home. Attention-deficit/hyperactivity disorder does not have to define who Denver is, but knowledge of it will allow his teachers and caregivers to learn how to support his dynamic brain as it develops over time.

Denver's parents want to know if his ADHD is mild or severe. Understanding symptom severity can help guide management decisions in terms of how quickly psychopharmacological treatment is pursued. A helpful resource for a potential clinical pathway for ADHD can be found online (www.chop.edu/clinical-pathway/adhd-clinical-pathway). The severity level of ADHD is based on the degree to which functioning is impaired but is somewhat subjective, as neurodivergent individuals' functioning can vary by skill, setting, and support over time.[13] Examples of different degrees of impairment at varying levels of ADHD severity could include

- **Mild:** speaking out of turn in the classroom, distracting classmates, losing assignments, not keeping track of deadlines
- **Moderate:** getting detention, being excluded from peer groups, facing declining grades because of missed work or work that has been rushed and contains incomplete work or mistakes despite knowing the information
- **Severe:** facing failing grades, getting suspended from school, withdrawing socially, avoiding school, getting kicked off a sports team

Based on these severity examples, Denver's ADHD is currently mild. Reassessment at follow-up visits is recommended, as the severity may change over time.

➤ **What can you suggest Denver's parents do at home and in partnership with the school to help manage his ADHD symptoms?**

Management: ADHD

- Support regulation and predictability through healthy routines.
  - — Encourage participation in structured sports or movement-based activities to help build team-based skills, build frustration tolerance, and increase ability to wait/take turns.
  - — Provide opportunities to build social skills with structured social skills groups or after-school activities.
  - — Encourage regular sleep, meals, and physical activity to support attention and emotion regulation.
  - — Limit screen time, particularly before bedtime.
  - — Provide consistent daily structure with clear, predictable routines and ample discussion when routines will change.
- Reduce stress and strengthen relationships.
  - — Schedule regular special time with parents that is child led, enjoyable, and free of correction or criticism.
  - — Emphasize and reflect the child's strengths, interests, and successes.
  - — Use calm, predictable responses to behavior to support a sense of safety.
- Psychosocial and skill-building interventions.
  - — Use positive reinforcement strategies such as reward systems, which focus on effort and building intrinsic motivation, rather than outcome and punishment.[14]
  - — Provide frequent praise for desired behaviors.[14]
  - — Seek social skills support groups to support peer relationships.[14]
  - — Seek organizational skills training to help enhance challenges in executive functioning and organization, particularly related to schoolwork.[14]
  - — Find additional emotion regulation skills training to help the child identify and manage frustration or sensory overloads.[14]
  - — Seek occupational therapy to help support integrated sensory development, including attention and executive functioning challenges, fine and gross motor coordination/handwriting, sitting still, and social skills.
- School-based supports and collaboration.
  - — Consider implementing a behavioral classroom management strategy (eg, a daily report card, frequent teacher or counselor check-ins).
  - — Increase parent-teacher contact and collaboration to create regular, collaborative communication between parents and teachers.[15]
  - — Seek educational supports such as a 504 plan or Individualized Education Program (IEP),[12,16] when appropriate, which focus on accommodations rather than discipline.

Keep in Mind: Neurodiversity

The concept of neurodiversity recognizes that human brains exhibit diverse characteristics, leading to variations in learning and cognitive processes. These variations are rooted in the inherent differences within the human brain. Attention-deficit/hyperactivity disorder is a neurodevelopmental disorder characterized by distinct brain development patterns.[2] These patterns undergo changes over time and can influence various aspects of an individual's behavior, social skills, communication abilities, cognitive functions, and motor coordination. Children with ADHD are considered neurodivergent, as they process information differently and exhibit a unique pace of development compared to their peers. In many ways, ADHD can be described as a superpower that needs to be harnessed because it has the potential to affect performance at school/home and in peer relationships.[6]

Denver's parents would like to know when starting a medication for his ADHD symptoms would be considered. In school-aged children, a medication can be considered for any severity of ADHD symptoms but is recommended when symptoms are moderate to severe and the medication is used alongside behavioral interventions. For youth 6 years and younger, the American Academy of Pediatrics (AAP) recommends Behavioral Parent Training (BPT) methods as a first-line approach to treatment before considering medication. For children older than 6 years, the AAP recommends combining medication treatment with behavioral interventions.[12] After a new diagnosis, establish a plan for regular follow-up and what criteria will be used to determine if adding medication to the management plan is warranted. Refer to Chapter 12, Attention-Deficit/Hyperactivity Disorder, for more information.

Back to the Case: Worsening Severity or a Coexisting Condition

Denver's parents worked with the school and obtained a 504 plan for him. As part of this plan, he received extended time on tests, a distraction-free testing environment, preferential seating in front of the teacher, and a daily report card with a reward system. At home, his parents limited his screen time, he joined a local soccer team, and he spent more time outside in his yard when not playing soccer. His parents created a nighttime routine and schedule for him and pinned it to a bulletin board in his room to help him independently move through the steps of getting ready for bed. Despite these interventions, Denver continued to struggle with some of his schoolwork. Throughout the academic year, his teacher noted that he had not made good progress in his English curriculum and his math grades had begun to decline. Denver has started to express frustration and say that he is stupid. His parents bring him to your office to see if his poor school performance is an indication that they should start medication for his ADHD.

Additional Differential Diagnosis: Worsening Severity or a Coexisting Condition

A declining school performance in a child with ADHD could indicate worsening severity of ADHD or a coexisting condition with ADHD. It could also indicate changes in the environment or other social history. Other diagnoses to consider include

- **Specific learning disorder:** Children may appear inattentive because of frustration with, lack of interest in, or limited ability in a school-related task. The inattention here will be reduced when the child is performing a skill that does not require them to use the affected cognitive process.[5]
  — For example, "He struggles with his math homework, but he has no problem remembering the rules in soccer." In one task, the demand requires reading comprehension and number processing, whereas in the other task, it requires auditory processing and working memory.
- **Anxiety disorder:** Children with an anxiety disorder can appear inattentive because of their preference to avoid anxiety-provoking activities or ruminate on worries.
- **Depression:** The inability to concentrate can be a symptom of a depressive episode.
- **Substance use disorder:** Less common at this age but can appear as inattention if the child is using substances that slow reaction time, slow processing speed, and interfere with working memory.
- **Sleep disorder:** Children with ADHD are at higher risk of having insomnia, circadian rhythm sleep-wake disorder, sleep-disordered breathing, and restless legs syndrome.[4,17]
- **Bullying:** Children who are being bullied at school can face academic struggles from being distracted or anxious during the school day.
- **Social factors:** Check for changes in environment such as people living in home, potential trauma, or other social conditions that could affect functioning.

Additional Evaluation: Worsening Severity or a Coexisting Condition

Because a pediatrician does not have firsthand observation of school performance, it will be important to have the family pursue a multidisciplinary team evaluation or psychoeducational evaluation either through the child's school or with a psychologist. Although ADHD is diagnosable by a pediatrician, there are benefits to these comprehensive evaluations, as they take a broader look into cognitive and academic development, in addition to looking into psychosocial functioning, executive functioning, and motor skills. At a minimum, obtaining school performance data will provide invaluable information to caregivers and pediatricians, who are not present during the school day.

Keep in Mind: School Collaborations

School-based partnerships are pivotal for the success of children with ADHD. Parents often actively engage in creating home-school collaboration, serving as mediators to facilitate communication with the medical team and obtaining the necessary rating scales for assessments and progress monitoring. However, if patients are experiencing difficulties in communicating with the school, it is essential to encourage them to make efforts to improve this relationship, as enhanced communication is beneficial for their academic success.[14,16]

Collaboration between school and the health care professional is also crucial. Pediatricians can collaborate with schools to comprehensively assess a child's functioning, and they can facilitate seamless communication and monitoring, thereby enhancing overall performance. The AAP *Caring for Children With ADHD: A Practical Resource Toolkit for Clinicians* contains information on strategies for managing ADHD in school settings. Additionally, the AAP website HealthyChildren.org has resources for parents about how schools can help children with ADHD (www.healthychildren.org/English/health-issues/conditions/adhd/Pages/default.aspx).

Back to the Case: Specific Learning Disorder

You help Denver's family advocate for a multidisciplinary evaluation (MDE), which is a comprehensive psychoeducational assessment that looks at academic, cognitive, and psychosocial functioning and behavior. This can often be done by drafting a letter requesting an MDE for the caregivers to sign and give to the school. If the family gets pushback from the school, you can tell them that they can insist on an evaluation or connect them with a resource coordinator such as a social worker or parent advocacy organization to help learn how to advocate for their child's educational rights. Since Denver is in a public school, this evaluation was completed by a school psychologist in his district and free of charge. Private providers such as psychologists and neuropsychologists can also perform this type of evaluation for a fee. Denver's multidisciplinary team evaluation demonstrated that in addition to ADHD, inattentive subtype, he also has an SLD, which is a neurodevelopmental disorder that affects processes related to reading, writing, and/or math.[5] His school is now developing an IEP and will be giving him access to other special education services to help him meet his academic goals.

Keep in Mind: Dyslexia

"Dyslexia" is used colloquially for learning disabilities but is an SLD subtype that refers to learning difficulties with word recognition, decoding, and spelling. Dyslexia alone does not include difficulties with reading comprehension or math reasoning.

➤ Does an evaluation for learning disabilities need to occur beyond what the school provides?

Multidisciplinary evaluations conducted by schools are typically sufficient for diagnosing learning disabilities. However, there are always providers outside school who can provide psychoeducational evaluations if additional testing is warranted. This testing may be expensive and may not be covered by insurance, so this can be a barrier for some families. Sometimes a neuropsychology evaluation will be covered by insurance if the child's cognitive concerns are thought to be attributable to another medical diagnosis, such as preterm birth or seizures, but this is insurance specific. It can be helpful to develop a list of psychologists or psychology evaluation clinics that can be provided to a caregiver if additional testing is requested.

Discussion: Specific Learning Disorder

Denver's parents ask, "Does having a specific learning disorder mean he isn't smart?"

For children with an SLD, the learning difficulties they experience are

- Below those expected for chronological age[5]
- Not better explained by intellectual developmental disorders (eg, intellectual disability, global developmental delay), hearing or vision disorders, or neurological or motor disorders[5]
- In individuals who otherwise demonstrate normal levels of intellectual functioning (generally estimated by IQ)[5]
- Not associated with general external factors, such as economic disadvantage, chronic absenteeism, or lack of education[5]
- In some individuals identified as intellectually gifted, sometimes referred to as being "twice exceptional"[5,17]

Having an SLD does not mean the child is not smart; rather, it identifies that there are some aspects of learning that are challenging. Further, a child with an SLD will greatly benefit from individualized learning adjustments through either an IEP or additional supports such as tutoring or academic learning centers.[18]

Specialized curricula for learning disabilities exist and are designed to help these students succeed academically. Examples include programs such as the Wilson Reading System for literacy development and Positive Action for social-emotional learning.

➤ What does an SLD have to do with mental health?

Individuals with learning challenges and disorders may present with behavioral concerns, such as reluctance to engage in academics, distractibility, or oppositional behaviors in response to learning demands. An SLD, however, is a common co-occurring condition of neurodevelopmental conditions (eg, ADHD, autism) and other mental health disorders (eg, anxiety and depressive disorders).[5,18] It is estimated that SLD coexists in approximately 45% of youth with ADHD; therefore, it is good practice to assess academic skills and performance deficits at the time of diagnosis.[19] If an SLD was not assessed for initially, it is important to evaluate anytime there is a change in academic performance because it can be challenging to know whether ADHD is contributing to academic challenges or if the contributor is an SLD.

➤ What is the difference between a 504 plan and an IEP?

Management: Specific Learning Disorder

A 504 plan is designated for students who do not qualify for special education services but have a disability that affects learning. Thus, a 504 plan creates accommodations such as classroom adjustments and curriculum modifications to help improve accessibility to the learning environment. An IEP is a specialized plan designed for students with disabilities as defined by the Individuals with Disabilities Education Act.[16] It customizes the curriculum to meet the unique needs of each student to receive optimal educational instruction. The accommodations in a 504 plan can be incorporated into an IEP if a student later qualifies for expanded services, as in the case with Denver. It is important to note that private and parochial schools do not have to follow IEPs or 504 plans and may not have the recommended services or accommodations available to offer.

Back to the Case: Continued Severity or Another Condition

The following summer, while attending a tennis day camp, Denver kicked another child, hit his racket against the net aggressively, and was thus dismissed from the summer camp. At home, he has been physically aggressive with his sister (eg, grabbing, pushing). He recently started third grade, and while the school has not yet noted issues, his parents are worried that his aggression may cause future disciplinary action at school. They bring him to your clinic and ask what could be causing the escalation of his aggressive behaviors.

Additional Differential Diagnosis: Aggression

- **Worsening symptoms of ADHD**
- **Adjustment disorder**
- **Anxiety**
- **Depression or bipolar disorder**
- **Posttraumatic stress disorder**
- **Trauma, including abuse**
- **Conduct disorder**
- **Disruptive mood dysregulation disorder (DMDD)**
- **Bereavement**
- **Sleep disturbance/disorder**
- **Bullying**
- **Malnutrition**
- **Lead exposure**
- **Pain/chronic pain**

There are a few key questions to ask to help identify what might be causing the change in Denver's behavior.

- Has there been a change in his social situation? Any identifiable social stressors? Any bullying?
- Are there any noticeable triggers to his aggressive acts?
  - — If so, are these triggers modifiable, such as improvement of sleep hygiene or removal from negative triggers, such as bullying or exposure to violence.

- What is his mood in between outbursts? Is he always irritable, frustrated, or impulsive, or is the mood episodic?
  - An irritable mood at baseline is more consistent with DMDD, whereas an episodically irritable mood is more consistent with ADHD.
- How much does he understand about his ADHD and learning issues?
  - As children mature, they can sometimes get angry or frustrated when they start to recognize that some tasks may be harder for them than their same-aged peers and, as such, may act out.
- How is his eating? Sleeping? Daily activity level?

Additional Evaluation: Aggression

- Consider readministering the NICHQ Vanderbilt Assessment Scale, which has a follow-up scale. The follow-up scale is intended to be used to monitor treatment progress and impairment level of symptoms and can be used periodically for this type of assessment. The full scale would need to be administered again if there is a prolonged gap in care, any new major changes, or new co-occurring symptoms.
- If the patient is taking an ADHD medication, ensure that the dosage is optimized for their age and weight.
- Check in on eating and sleeping habits.
- Collect input from the parents, teacher, coach, or therapist, or any other adults who might have insight into this behavioral change.
- Obtain updated social history, including stressors, trauma, bullying, screen time, or life changes.

Additional screening and assessment tools to consider, as linked to and further detailed in the Appendix, include

- **Strengths and Difficulties Questionnaire (SDQ):** A general behavioral screening questionnaire, for children and adolescents aged 2 to 17 years, that focuses on emotional symptoms, conduct, hyperactivity/impulsivity, peer relationships, and prosocial behavioral concerns. The questionnaire can flag areas of concern and prosocial strengths.
  - 25 items; can be completed by parents, teachers, or child (age dependent)
- **Pediatric Symptom Checklist-17 (PSC-17):** Widely used parent-completed measure of a child's psychosocial functioning, normed for children and adolescents aged 4 to 17 years, including internalized problems (eg, anxiety, depression), attention issues, and externalizing problems (eg, disruptive and oppositional behaviors). This is a briefer version of the PSC-35. Refer to Chapter 5, Somatic Symptoms and Depression, for additional details.

- **Screen for Child Anxiety and Related Emotional Disorders (SCARED):** A pediatric anxiety screener used for children 8 years and older. A total score of 25 or higher may indicate the presence of an anxiety disorder. Child and parent rating scale versions are available.
  — Additionally, this screener will give the clinician subscale scores, which may indicate a specific type of anxiety disorder such as generalized anxiety disorder, social anxiety disorder, panic, school anxiety, and separation anxiety.

Discussion: Aggression

Attention-deficit/hyperactivity disorder is characterized by a lack of impulse control, hyperactivity, and/or persistent inattention.[4] Consequently, children with ADHD may experience difficulties in decision-making or do things that result in disciplinary problems or social difficulties. Children with ADHD may also encounter challenges in emotion regulation and communication, which can complicate the management of impulses, anger, and frustration. When confronted with criticism, judgment, or misunderstanding, children with ADHD may be prone to experiencing anger and subsequently act without fully considering the potential consequences.

Anger reactions can also be linked to self-esteem concerns.[20] As children with ADHD mature, they may come to realize that certain activities are more challenging than others. This realization can lead to frustration and subsequently trigger an anger response.

As children age, expectations from parents and teachers also increase, which can lead to increased stress. Children may also spend more time in settings where accommodations are unavailable, such as sports or camps, which may result in emotional dysregulation.

Management: Aggression

- Emotion regulation training.
- Improve communication skills and seek speech therapy if there is an underlying communication deficit.
- Parenting program[14] (refer also to a helpful online resource: "Evidence-Based Psychosocial Interventions for ADHD" [www.chop.edu/clinical-pathway/adhd-care-evidence-based-psychosocial-interventions]).
  — Behavioral Parent Training/Parent Management Training (BPT/PMT)
  — The Incredible Years
  — Positive Parenting Program (Triple P)
  — Parent-Child Interaction Therapy (PCIT)
  — Helping the Noncompliant Child parent training program

- Optimize ADHD medication management (refer to Chapter 12, Attention-Deficit/ Hyperactivity Disorder).
- Consider adding an α_2-adrenergic agonist (refer to Chapter 12, Attention-Deficit/ Hyperactivity Disorder).

Keep in Mind: Caregiving Strategies for Behavioral Challenges

Caregivers of children with behavioral challenges associated with ADHD may feel they spend most of their time focusing on maladaptive behaviors and acting as a disciplinarian. It is important to help guide them in rebuilding a healthy, positive relationship with their child. Here are a few strategies.

- Focus on the positive. Remember that children with ADHD probably get critiqued and hear negative feedback all day long. Try to ignore minor infractions and focus on the positive whenever possible.
- Set kids up for success. Minimize potential triggers such as quick transitions and prolonged screen time without limits, and optimize sleep, nutrition, and exercise.
- Remain calm and consistent.
- Try talking less! Make statements and commands brief and simple.
- Create a safety plan. Make the home a safe place for the child and develop a plan for what will happen if negative behaviors escalate. Keep emergency numbers in your phone and reach out to your child's pediatric clinician for help.

Conclusion

Attention-deficit/hyperactivity disorder and specific learning disorder often co-occur and can complicate the diagnosis of each because of symptom/ behavior overlap.[21] Patients with each of these diagnoses are at risk for significant challenges in school, and this is compounded by having both diagnoses, as is the risk for coexisting mental health diagnoses. Therefore, it is important to complete a comprehensive assessment and continue to regularly reassess the patient anytime there is a behavior or academic change, to ensure that appropriate psychosocial interventions and supports are in place to optimize academic performance and social functioning as a child grows.

Lessons Learned From the Tornado

In the Tornado case (as ADHD and learning difficulties unfold), the child may exhibit chaotic energy that feels relentless, but with proper psychosocial support, parent and child behavior management, and potential targeted medication, symptoms can be mitigated to reduce frustration, impulsivity, and aggression.

- Attention-deficit/hyperactivity disorder can present with inattention, hyperactivity, or both.
- ADHD can look different across different time points as the brain matures.[7]
- Attention-deficit/hyperactivity disorder and learning disorders are highly comorbid and can make school very challenging.[4,5]
- Learning disorders can present with behavioral symptoms.
- Learning disorders can include an impairment in reading, written expression, and/or math, but when specifically characterized by problems with word recognition, decoding, or spelling ability, they may be called "dyslexia."[5]
- Learning disorders are not a sign of lower intelligence but rather a representation of academic functioning that does not correspond to the expected performance based on age, opportunity, and intelligence.[5]
- Children with ADHD and learning disorders may be eligible for an IEP, which can provide specialized education if necessary, or a 504 plan, which can offer accommodations to support their educational performance.[16]
- Aggression can be a manifestation of poor impulse control from ADHD and may benefit from first optimizing ADHD management.[22]
- There is strong evidence to support behavioral and parent training interventions for children with ADHD, as well as medication.[12,14,21]

Keywords: ADHD, aggression, dyslexia, learning disability, poor school performance, specific learning disorder, Vanderbilt scales

Suggested Reading

Barbaresi WJ, Campbell L, Diekroger EA, et al. Society for Developmental and Behavioral Pediatrics clinical practice guideline for the assessment and treatment of children and adolescents with complex attention-deficit/hyperactivity disorder. *J Dev Behav Pediatr*. 2020;41:S35–S57 PMID: 31996577

Kates MS, LaFreniere LS. School-based interventions for attention-deficit/hyperactivity disorder (ADHD) in middle schools: a review of the literature. *Educ Sci*. 2025;15(9):1225

Pham AV, Riviere A. Specific learning disorders and ADHD: current issues in diagnosis across clinical and educational settings. *Curr Psychiatry Rep*. 2015;17(6):38 PMID: 25894357

References

1. American Psychiatric Association. Other neurodevelopmental disorders. In: *Diagnostic and Statistical Manual of Mental Disorders*. 5th ed, text rev. American Psychiatric Association Publishing; 2022:99
2. American Psychiatric Association. Oppositional defiant disorder. In: *Diagnostic and Statistical Manual of Mental Disorders*. 5th ed, text rev. American Psychiatric Association Publishing; 2022:523–527
3. Gomez R, Stavropoulos V, Gomez A, Brown T, Watson S. Network analyses of oppositional defiant disorder (ODD) symptoms in children. *BMC Psychiatry*. 2022;22(1):263 PMID: 35418047
4. American Psychiatric Association. Attention-deficit/hyperactivity disorder. In: *Diagnostic and Statistical Manual of Mental Disorders*. 5th ed, text rev. American Psychiatric Association Publishing; 2022:69–76
5. American Psychiatric Association. Specific learning disorder. In: *Diagnostic and Statistical Manual of Mental Disorders*. 5th ed, text rev. American Psychiatric Association Publishing; 2022:76
6. Eide B, Eide F. *The Dyslexic Advantage: Unlocking the Hidden Potential of the Dyslexic Brain*. Rev and updated ed. Plume; 2023
7. Tremblay S, Willcutt EG. Implications of co-occurrence between ADHD and anxiety in a community-based child sample. *J Atten Disord*. 2025;29(11):911–923 PMID: 40130654
8. American Psychiatric Association. Delirium. In: *Diagnostic and Statistical Manual of Mental Disorders*. 5th ed, text rev. American Psychiatric Association Publishing; 2022:672–674
9. Duffee J, Szilagyi M, Forkey H, Kelly ET; American Academy of Pediatrics Council on Community Pediatrics; Council on Foster Care, Adoption, and Kinship Care; Council on Child Abuse and Neglect; and Committee on Psychosocial Aspects of Child and Family Health. Trauma-informed care in child health systems. *Pediatrics*. 2021;148(2):e2021052580 PMID: 34312294
10. Forkey H, Szilagyi M, Kelly ET, Duffee J; American Academy of Pediatrics Council on Foster Care, Adoption, and Kinship Care; Council on Community Pediatrics; Council on Child Abuse and Neglect; and Committee on Psychosocial Aspects of Child and Family Health. Trauma-informed care. *Pediatrics*. 2021;148(2):e2021052581 PMID: 34312292
11. American Academy of Pediatrics Council on Environmental Health. Prevention of childhood lead toxicity. *Pediatrics*. 2016;138(1):e20161493 PMID: 27325637

12. Wolraich ML, Hagan JF Jr, Allan C, et al; American Academy of Pediatrics Subcommittee on Children and Adolescents With Attention-Deficit/Hyperactive Disorder. Clinical practice guideline for the diagnosis, evaluation, and treatment of attention-deficit/hyperactivity disorder in children and adolescents. *Pediatrics*. 2019;144(4):e20192528 PMID: 31570648
13. Gillette H. Why we no longer say high or low functioning for autism. Healthline. December 12, 2023. Accessed March 23, 2026. https://www.healthline.com/health/autism/functioning-labels-autism
14. Lockwood K; Children's Hospital of Philadelphia. *Primary Care Perspectives*. ADHD treatment: how psychosocial interventions can be used with children and adolescents. April 17, 2025. Accessed May 26, 2026. https://www.podbean.com/media/share/pb-yxud7-1883a65
15. Mautone JA, Marshall SA, Sharman J, Eiraldi RB, Jawad AF, Power TJ. Development of a family-school intervention for young children with attention deficit hyperactivity disorder. *School Psych Rev*. 2012;41(4):447–466 PMID: 24353368
16. Individuals with Disabilities Education Act, 20 USC §1400 (2004)
17. Arky B. Twice-exceptional kids: both gifted and challenged. Child Mind Institute. December 18, 2025. Accessed March 23, 2026. https://childmind.org/article/twice-exceptional-kids-both-gifted-and-challenged
18. Frankowski BL. Learning difficulty. In: Foy JM, ed. *Mental Health Care of Children and Adolescents: A Guide for Primary Care Clinicians*. American Academy of Pediatrics; 2018:600–615
19. DuPaul GJ, Gormley MJ, Laracy SD. Comorbidity of LD and ADHD: implications of *DSM-5* for assessment and treatment. *J Learn Disabil*. 2013;46(1):43–51 PMID: 23144063
20. Lök N, Bademli K, Canbaz M. The effects of anger management education on adolescents' manner of displaying anger and self-esteem: a randomized controlled trial. *Arch Psychiatr Nurs*. 2018;32(1):75–81 PMID: 29413078
21. Wissow LS. Inattention and impulsivity. In: Foy JM, ed. *Mental Health Care of Children and Adolescents: A Guide for Primary Care Clinicians*. American Academy of Pediatrics; 2018:585–599
22. Saylor KE, Amann BH. Impulsive aggression as a comorbidity of attention-deficit/hyperactivity disorder in children and adolescents. *J Child Adolesc Psychopharmacol*. 2016;26(1):19–25 PMID: 26744906

CHAPTER 9

Suicidality and Eating Disorder

The Snowball: A representation of what was, characterized by withering away, sadness, and disappearing. Look out for isolation, self-harm, or thoughts of death.

Presentation

Savannah, a 15-year-old, has been taking escitalopram, a selective serotonin reuptake inhibitor (SSRI), for 5 weeks. You prescribed the medication after following up with her for mild depression for the past year and noting that her symptom severity had worsened in the past 3 months. At the time of SSRI initiation, you discussed the black box warning and had Savannah start with a low dose (5 mg). At the 3-week follow-up visit, Savannah had no adverse effects from the escitalopram, so you increased her dose to 10 mg. She returns to you 2 weeks later with suicidal ideation.

Savannah reports that she has started to have some thoughts of not wanting to be here anymore. When she woke up today, she thought, "Is this my life; is this all there is?" Later, when she was in art class, while using a cutting tool, she thought, "I could use this to cut myself," and imagined blood. You asked her what stopped her from carrying out this act and she said, "It seemed like it would be dramatic for school." Savannah didn't tell anyone about these thoughts until she arrived at your office.

Patient History

- **Medical history:** Prior generalized anxiety disorder (diagnosed at age 11 years) and depression (diagnosed 1 year ago).
- **Mental health care:** Has been seeing a therapist for 1 year.
- **Family history:** Her mom has a history of anxiety; her maternal grandmother has a history of depression while taking escitalopram.
- **Social history (using the SSHADESS framework)**
  - — **S**trengths: Art.
  - — **S**chool: Is an average student (Bs), but lately has had some Cs.
  - — **H**ome: Her parents divorced when she was 10 years old. She splits time between parents' homes. Her mom has a new boyfriend, and her dad remarried 3 years ago. She does not like her stepmother; she has a stepsister who is 15 years old.
  - — **A**ctivities: Art club after school once a week.
  - — **D**rugs: She responds that she does not use alcohol, tobacco products, or marijuana.
  - — **E**motions: She had generalized anxiety disorder, but she has been able to manage her anxiety symptoms well for the past few years. In the past year, her mood became increasingly sad, so she started to see a therapist. Despite therapy, her sad mood has worsened. She reports that stressors in her life are related to her parents' divorce and not liking splitting time between households with different rules. Does not eat well at her mom's house and has more bouts of crying while there. Trouble sleeping at both houses and sometimes uses melatonin for sleep.
  - — **S**exuality: Attracted to males; no sexual activity.
  - — **S**afety: Feels safe at home and school; no bullying; no guns in either home; has not been in any fights; no history of physical or sexual abuse.
- **Medication:** Escitalopram taken at 10 mg daily.

➤ **What are some known risk factors for suicidal ideation in patients?**

Risk Factors

- Behavioral or emotional concerns, including depression
- Positive findings on depression screening, such as the Patient Health Questionnaire-9 Modified for Adolescents (PHQ-A) or Ask Suicide-Screening Questions (ASQ)
- Chronic or acute medical illness
- A decline in overall functioning, whether in activities of daily living, school performance, social engagement, or medical treatment adherence
- Recent suicidal ideation or behavior, including self-harm
- Early life adversity[1]

Suicidal behaviors include (from least to most severe)

- Preparatory acts: gathering pills, writing a suicide note
- Aborted attempt or self-interrupted attempt: stops because of the patient's own decision
- Interrupted attempt: stops because of outside circumstances
- Actual attempt: an act carried out for the purpose of dying

➤ **How would you assess a patient's suicidal ideation in terms of severity?**

Evaluation

One empirically supported method to assess for suicidality is using a screening tool such as the Columbia-Suicide Severity Rating Scale (C-SSRS).[2,3] The C-SSRS is a clinically validated screening tool used to assess suicidal ideation and behavior.[2] Refer to the Appendix for a link to the tool online. It can also provide information on severity, plan, and immediate risk/intent.[3] Suicidality occurs on a spectrum, which ranges from

- Wish for death: "Have you wished you were dead or wished you could go to sleep and not wake up?"
- Suicidal ideation: "Have you had any thoughts of killing or hurting yourself?"
- Suicidal ideation with method: "If so, have you thought about how you might do it?"
- Suicidal ideation with intent: "When you've had these thoughts, do you think you'll actually act on it or do it?"
- Suicidal ideation with intent and plan: "Have you thought about how you would hurt or kill yourself?"
- Suicidal behavior: "Have you ever done anything before to hurt or try to end your life?"

Severity (acuity) can be graded by what type of suicidal ideation the patient has experienced in the past month.[3]

- Low acuity → wish for death
- Intermediate acuity → suicidal ideation or suicidal ideation with method but not intent, plan, or behavior
- High acuity → suicidal ideation with intent or plan, or suicidal behavior

Keep in Mind: A Conversation About Suicidal Ideation

Assessing for suicidal ideation can be difficult and requires sensitivity and empathy. One of the benefits of using a screening tool such as the C-SSRS is that the questions are created in plain language and can be used conversationally. Given the sensitive nature of asking suicide-related questions, it is important to take ample time to ask the questions and listen to the responses, treating the exchange more like a conversation then a checklist of questions to complete. Clinicians should remain calm and consider themselves in a place of privilege that the patient is choosing to share this with them and that they are now in a position to offer help.

For patients at risk for suicide, a helpful clinical pathway for assessment and care planning can be found online (www.chop.edu/clinical-pathway/suicide-risk-assessment-and-care-planning-clinical-pathway).

In this case, Savannah expresses suicidal ideation ("Is this my life; is this all there is?") and identifies a method (cutting self with tool). It would be important to further evaluate whether she had intent or a plan. To assess this, the clinician could ask

- **Intent:** "When you had those thoughts about cutting your skin with a tool, did you think you'd do it?" or "Have you ever felt like you might act on those thoughts to end your life?"
- **Plan:** "Have you thought about how you would end your life?" "Have you ever made a plan for how you might hurt yourself or even kill yourself?" "Have you ever gathered things you need (eg, pills, knives) that you'd use?" or "Have you written a note to anyone in preparation for killing yourself?"

➤ Which screening tools could you use to assess depression severity in a patient?

Screening tools to assess the severity of Savannah's suicidal ideation include the PHQ-A and ASQ.[4–6] Refer to the Appendix for links to the tools online.

- **Patient Health Questionnaire-9 Modified for Adolescents (PHQ-A):** A depression screening tool for youth aged 11 to 17 years. The PHQ-A consists of 8 items that help classify differences in levels of depressive symptoms and 1 item related to suicidal ideation (eg, "Thoughts that you would be better off dead, or of hurting yourself in some way?"). It can be a helpful tool when assessing for anxiety, as the 2 disorders are highly comorbid. It can also serve as a symptom tracker and progress-monitoring tool if used over time.
  - Cutoff scores are
    - 5—mild
    - 10—moderate
    - 15—moderately severe
    - 20—severe
  - If suicidal ideation is endorsed, it requires immediate follow-up with a more investigative suicide screener, such as the ASQ or C-SSRS; safety planning; and referral for external support.
- **Ask Suicide-Screening Questions (ASQ):** Suicide risk screening tool; validated for youth 10 years and older, but can be used for children as young as 8 years.
  - 4 questions; a response of "Yes" to at least 1 is identified as a suicide risk.
  - The American Academy of Pediatrics (AAP) recommends universal suicide screening for youth 12 years and older.

In this case, Savannah's PHQ-A score is available from an earlier visit, so it makes sense to readminister the PHQ-A and use the C-SSRS to quantitatively measure how her symptoms have changed since the previous assessment. Refer to Table 9–1 for scores.

Table 9–1. Savannah's PHQ-A and C-SSRS Scores

Items	Range	Score (Classification)
Total PHQ-A score on questions 1–8	0–27	27 (severe depression)
PHQ-A score on question 9 (suicide risk)	1–4	3 (SUICIDE RISK)
C-SSRS—clinically significant	24	Wish to be dead: Yes Non-specific active suicidal thoughts: Yes Active suicidal ideation with any methods (not plan) without intent to act: Yes Active suicidal ideation with some intent to act, without specific plan: No Active suicidal ideation with specific plan and intent: No

Abbreviations: C-SSRS, Columbia-Suicide Severity Rating Scale; PHQ-A, Patient Health Questionnaire-9 Modified for Adolescents.

Keep in Mind: Passive Versus Active Suicidal Ideation

In practice, there is usually a distinction between "passive" suicidal ideation, where there is no plan or intent to kill oneself (eg, "I wish I could go to sleep and never wake up") and "active" suicidal ideation, which implies active plan, behaviors, or intent (eg, "I don't see the point in living anymore and wanted to jump in front of the train this morning to just end it all"). More recent practice suggests moving away from these categorial terms, as the passive category may minimize risk and reduce the urgency to assess further and act. Current terminology suggests using the word *general* to describe death wishes without plan or intent and to consider suicidality as more of a spectrum.

When Savannah's previous and current PHQ-A scores are compared, they show that her depression has moved from moderately severe to severe and that there is now a risk for suicide.

••• Communication Pearl •••
Discussing Suicidal Ideation With Families

For some caregivers, the first time they hear about their child's suicidal ideation is in the clinic setting. Give them time to process this news. Ask follow-up questions, such as "What was it like for you to hear that?" Help families understand and contextualize their child's thoughts. Explain that while general thoughts can be common, acts are not, and that suicidal ideation is often an indicator of other mental health concerns. Suicidal thoughts that occur with a specific plan, intention, or method are more concerning. Offer support in whatever way you can and schedule a follow-up with the family to confirm that they make a linkage to treatment with a mental health specialist.

➤ Does Savannah have any known risk factors for suicide?

Risk factors for suicide to consider for Savannah include being female (as females have a higher risk of suicidal ideation and attempts), being 15 years or older (as teenagers have developmental and biological changes that affect mood, emotion regulation, and sensitivity to social stress/peer issues), having comorbid depression, and experiencing psychosocial stressors.[6–10] According to the Guidelines for Adolescent Depression in Primary Care, other risk factors to consider in history taking include previous attempts, substance use disorder, psychosis, lack of social supports, organized plan, no significant other/confidant, and first-degree relative who died by suicide.[6]

In addition, risk factors for suicide and suicidal ideation include social drivers of health, such as racism, discrimination, economic instability, and exposure to adverse childhood experiences, including abuse, neglect, and bullying.[11] Approximately 45% of LGBTQIA+ youth have had suicidal ideation and 14% have attempted suicide.[12,13] In one systematic review and meta-analysis, approximately 25% of patients with autism spectrum disorder had suicidal ideation.[14] Racial, ethnic, and gender minorities are more likely to face marginalization, which creates stress and places them at greater risk for suicidal ideation.[15] About 18% of youth with suicidal ideation make a suicide plan.[16]

➤ How do you assess Savannah's risk for suicide?

It is important to complete a brief suicide safety assessment (BSSA). The AAP has resources for conducting a BSSA on its website (www.aap.org/en/patient-care/blueprint-for-youth-suicide-prevention/strategies-for-clinical-settings-for-youth-suicide-prevention/conducting-a-brief-suicide-safety-assessment).

1. **PLAN:** Does she have a plan? If so, what method has she chosen? How likely is this method to kill her? What are her expectations of this method to kill her?
   - In this case, Savannah said she thought about cutting herself with a razor blade. She has access to this cutting tool daily in her art class, and similar tools are kept in her home. A strategic cut with this blade could kill her, and Savannah seems to understand this possibility.
2. **INTENT:** How strong is her intent to die? Has she thought about what would happen if she did die? Did she tell anyone about her suicidal thoughts, or would she tell anyone if they happened again? Does she identify ambivalence about living, or does she express hope?
   - In this case, her intent to die is not strong, but she did start thinking about what would happen if she died. Also, she did not immediately tell anyone about her suicidal thoughts. The clinician should ask her if she would tell anyone, should she have these thoughts again, and assess that person's ability to intervene/respond.
3. **SAFETY:** Can she be kept safe? This includes having a safe home, having supervision, not using substances, and being able to do self-care.
   - **Safe home:** The most common cause of suicide in teens is suffocation (mostly hanging), followed by guns and poisoning. Parents or caregivers need to be able to remove ropes, cables, guns, and weapons from the home. Other potentially harmful items include sharp knives, razor blades, alcohol, drugs, medications, and poisons.
   - **Supervision:** Can the parent/caregiver regularly check in with the youth about thoughts of suicide? Can they also identify suicidal behaviors (eg, expressing self-destructive thoughts, drawing morbid pictures, listening to music and watching media centered on themes of death, playing violent video games, giving away possessions).

- **Substance use:** Does the youth drink alcohol? Use drugs? Parents may be unaware of this behavior, so this is something the clinician should encourage the patient to talk about with their parent so it can be monitored and access to alcohol can be prevented.
- **Self-care:** Doing physical activity, having healthy nutrition, spending time with people who support them, relaxing, scheduling pleasant activities (behavioral activation), and setting small goals and simple steps.

4. **PROTECTIVE FACTORS:** What has kept her safe so far? What would stop her from acting on these thoughts if she had them again? Who are the people that love her and would miss her if she were to harm herself?

Keep in Mind: Black Box Warning

In a US Food and Drug Administration (FDA)–pooled analysis of 24 studies, the relative risk of suicidality posed is 2 times greater for SSRIs compared to placebo (ie, 2% risk with placebo, 4% risk with medication).[17] There were no deaths by suicide in any of the studies.

Clinicians should discuss the black box warning for SSRIs at the time of prescribing. However, emphasize with caregivers that prior studies showed an increase in suicidal thoughts but not acts.[17] Children and adolescents with untreated depression are also at risk for suicide.[6,17] During initiation of SSRIs, close monitoring for suicidality is important and should be done by both prescriber and caregivers.

Back to the Case: Suicidal Ideation

Savannah's parents ask if the escitalopram is causing her suicidal ideation because it seemed to begin 5 weeks after starting escitalopram and 2 weeks after a dosage increase.

Untreated depression is a risk factor for suicide.[6] When starting an SSRI in a patient, clinicians should weigh the risks and benefits of using an SSRI for that individual patient. In this case, in addition to reviewing her prior PHQ-A results, the clinician can ask Savannah if she recalls having suicidal ideation before she began taking escitalopram or if these thoughts developed after taking the medication. This is another indicator of how important it is for clinicians to use suicidal ideation screening tools to establish a baseline when initiating an SSRI so they have information to compare moving forward.

Knowing that her untreated moderate depression is its own risk factor for suicide, you come to a mutual decision with the patient and her parents that you should continue to titrate her SSRI dose to 15 mg. Moderate depression is best treated initially with evidence-based psychotherapy in combination with an SSRI, like fluoxetine or escitalopram. [6,18] Additionally, you work with Savannah's parents to create a suicide safety plan.

➤ **What is a suicide safety plan?**

Management: Suicidal Ideation

The next step in care is to create a suicide safety plan to ensure that Savannah is safe to go home. This is a collaboratively created plan to avoid suicide, seek support, and create a safe environment. One plan often used and adapted into clinical practice is called the **Stanley-Brown Safety Plan,** which helps identify warning signs/triggers, coping signs, and safe plans for suicidal thoughts and behaviors.[7,19] Please note, preferred language about these tools is *plans* and not *contracts*. Contracts imply a binding agreement that might prove hard for patient adherence in true suicidal crises and could lead to feelings of failure or judgment in those events. The goal is to create a written document that covers 6 topics with fill-in-the-blank sections for answers (Table 9-2). This document should ideally be printed and given to the patient to take home. It can also be documented in the file/health record for continuity of care with proper privacy conditions in place.

Table 9-2. Example of a Suicide Safety Plan

Steps	Description	Example of Patient Response
1. Warning Signs	Thoughts, images, moods, or behaviors that might be signs of a crisis developing	When I find out that I'm left out of a group text and feel like my friends are having fun without me
2. Internal Coping Strategies	Things I can do to take my mind off my problems without contacting another person	I can listen to music or take my dog for a walk in the park.
3. Social Contacts and Distractions	People and social settings that provide distraction	I can call my cousin or talk with my teacher at school.
4. People to Ask for Help	Typically, trusted adults who can provide help and support	My parents or my school counselor
5. Professionals and Crisis Resources	Professionals or professional services I can contact during a crisis	Dial 988 or 1-800-274-TALK (8255).
6. Making the Environment Safer	Safety plan for lethal means	Locking up pills and putting away sharp objects, like knives

Because firearms are currently the leading cause of death in children, the AAP recommends a multipronged approach focused on harm reduction, which includes safer firearm storage and lethal means counseling for patients and families with individuals at risk for self-harm and suicide. Safer-storage counseling includes telling caregivers that their firearm should be stored unloaded, locked, separate from the ammunition, and with the ammunition also locked. This counseling should be included along with other environmental safety measures including safe medication storage and removal of sharp objects.[20]

Savannah splits time between both parents' homes, so you must ensure that the safety plan can be followed in each home environment. Educate the patient and family about the 988 Lifeline, the free national mental health hotline, which has options to call, text, or chat with a counselor who can provide emotional support and assistance to individuals experiencing distress. While the patient and family are in the clinic, suggest they add the number to their phones (1-800-274-TALK [8255]).

After creating the safety plan, it is good practice to make a copy for the patient's health record as well as one for the patient's home. It is also important to think about parental involvement. If the child is younger, it is generally recommended to include the parent in the entire safety plan. With adolescents, use clinical judgment for steps 1 through 5, but it is strongly encouraged to have a parent or guardian be present when conducting step 6 (Making the Environment Safer).

➤ What is the best way to determine if a patient is safe to go home or should be transferred to the emergency department for further evaluation?

At the end of the clinical session, it is important to consider if the patient is safe to go home or if an immediate higher level of care is warranted. Use the obtained screening tools along with clinical assessment of severity and the documented safety plan to decide if further action is required.

- Is the patient at current risk for attempted or death by suicide?
- Are the family and patient able to adhere to recommendations about safety, supervision, and follow-up care?

Indications for hospitalization include

- Intent to die
- Suicide attempt
- Specific plan that is well conceived and potentially fatal
  - — Plan is feasible in youth's environment.
- Access to lethal means
- Significant risk factors (ie, previous attempts, severe depression, substance use, exposure to recent suicide by a loved one)
- Altered mental status
- Lack of social support to stay safe

If a patient is not willing to participate in outpatient treatment or does not have caregivers who can provide appropriate support, supervision, safety planning, and follow-up, then outpatient care may not be the safest option and this may also be an indication for hospitalization. Take a moment to consider the appropriate level of care (Figure 9-1), and if unsure about outpatient support, seek guidance from a trained mental health specialist. Above all, it is important to take a collaborative care approach in which communication occurs across multiple providers and places, including primary care physicians, schools, emergency departments, mental health specialists, and other community resources.

Figure 9-1. Mental Health Care Arranged From Lowest Entry Point of Contact to Highest Level of Intervention

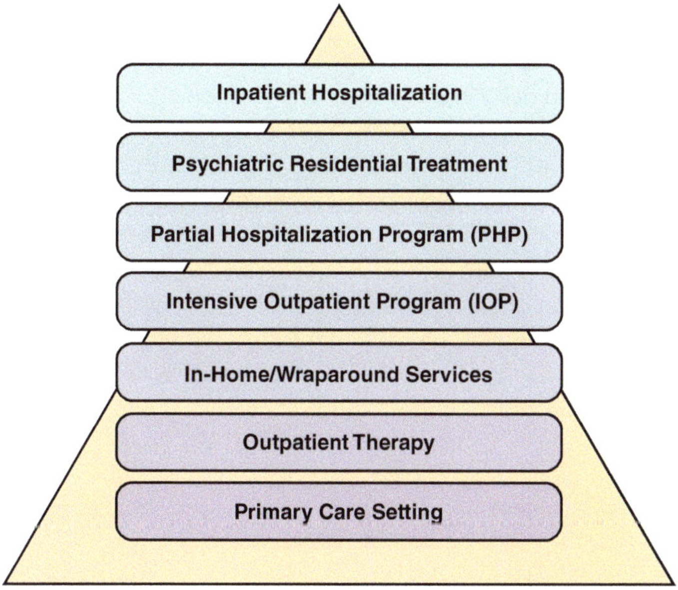

If acuity of the patient is deemed safe for outpatient therapy, there are a few evidence-based therapies that can be recommended for the outpatient.[21] These include

- Cognitive behavioral therapy, including cognitive behavioral therapy for suicide prevention (CBT-SP),[22] integrated cognitive behavioral therapy (I-CBT), family-based cognitive behavioral therapy,[23] and internet-based cognitive behavioral therapy (iCBT)[24,25]
- Dialectical behavior therapy for adolescents (DBT-A)[26,27]: for adolescents with self-harm, suicidal ideation, and emotional dysregulation
- Attachment-based family therapy (ABFT)

Keep in Mind: Technology and Intervention

Recent advances in technology, along with teenage comfort with screens, has led to research on how technology can help address more acute mental health crises like suicide. Telehealth and smartphone apps are 2 platforms that are becoming widely studied and used for their accessibility and scalability in terms of treatment outreach.[28,29] Telehealth has been shown to improve outcomes in medical settings, especially when emergency assessments are warranted or timely access to support is limited. It can provide access to medication management, clinical check-ins, and peer consultation.

Back to the Case: Non-Suicidal Self Injury

Savannah follows up closely over the next few months with both you and her therapist. She continues taking escitalopram at 15 mg, and her PHQ-A scores are trending down slightly to the 10 to 14 (moderate) range. She no longer endorses suicidal ideation. However, during a follow-up visit with her, you note linear superficial lacerations on her wrists. When talking confidentially with you, she reports that she has been cutting herself with a razor blade at home but only to relieve stress and that she does not have any intent to end her life. Savannah says she has a friend who cuts, and she learned cutting from her. She wears sweatshirts to cover up the marks, so her family and teachers haven't noticed.

➤ **Is cutting a form of suicidal ideation?**

Discussion: Non-Suicidal Self-Injury

Savannah is exhibiting non-suicidal self-injury (NSSI), which can be a form of suicidal ideation. Consisting of behaviors such as cutting, burning, and doing things that may cause pain but without the intent to die, it is often described as a coping mechanism to deal with stress or emotional pain, and the act and subsequent pain can be described as a physical and emotional "release."[30,31] Self-injury can sometimes be a precursor to suicide and should therefore be addressed in a serious manner.[31,32] Research suggests that NSSI, like cutting, may reduce a person's natural inhibition to hurt their own body over time. Therefore, people can become desensitized to thoughts of harm and self-inflicted pain, which can lead to the potential for more lethal actions.

The C-SSRS includes questions about self-injury, but if a clinician is not using a specific screening tool, it is always important for them to assess for NSSI. The clinician could use a question such as "You've said you do not wish to die, but sometimes people do things to their bodies like cutting their skin. Have you ever done anything like that?" It is important for youth to understand there is no safe form of cutting.

➤ When should a clinician break confidentiality with their adolescent patient?

It is developmentally appropriate for adolescents to build autonomy, and this includes making medical decisions. Legally, they are typically granted the right to consent to care related to specific health issues, including substance use and mental health, although the ages at which this right is granted, and when parental notification is required, vary from state to state.[33] Therefore, it is important to be aware of the local state and federal laws regarding minor confidentiality and safety in the area where you practice.

Encouraging adolescents to share information with their parents, even when not legally required, encourages communication and relationship building between the adolescent and parent. Having both the adolescent and the parent sharing knowledge that affects your clinical care can also help improve clinical outcomes.[33] Disclosing suicidal ideation or NSSI may be a difficult conversation for the adolescent, but the pediatric clinician can offer to help the adolescent navigate this conversation with their parents. If a patient is hesitant and not ready, and their thoughts and behaviors are not posing an immediate safety risk, the clinician can offer talking with the parents/guardian for the patient or think about including them in a conversation in the future. For example, the clinician can say, "I think it's important to let your parents know about your cutting to keep you safe and so they can support you. We don't have to give them all the details and can share the talking responsibilities, but I think it can be helpful." If an adolescent is not disclosing NSSI to their parent, it is also important to let them know that this could change if their behaviors change and if you have any new safety concerns. Understanding the limits of confidentiality is important so that an adolescent does not feel like their trust was violated if you need to break confidentiality later on and so that any potential negative effect on the pediatrician-patient relationship can be minimized.[33]

Back to the Case: Depression Remission

A year has passed, and Savannah's depression has improved, with PHQ-A scores in the 0 to 4 range (none/mild). She no longer has self-injurious behaviors. She feels therapy has helped, and her family has been more engaged and present with her, which she has really enjoyed. She has been attending art club once a week after school and hangs out with friends on the weekends. Savannah would like to wean off her escitalopram, and her parents agree with trying this.

➤ How do you determine if your patient's depression is in remission?

Management: Depression Remission

Given that Savannah no longer has a low mood, her PHQ-A scores have decreased, and her NSSI has ceased, Savannah no longer meets criteria for depression based on your screening and assessment. Depression is considered in remission when criteria are no longer met and there is an increase in social, emotional, physical, and cognitive functioning. Depression can be considered in full remission if the improvement has been noted for more than 2 months or partial remission if it has lasted less time but the patient shows a reduction in symptom criteria with an ability to return to baseline functioning in school and home life.[1,6]

Keep in Mind: "Curing" Depression

Generally, depression is considered a recurring condition, meaning that it is likely that a person will have another episode in their lifetime.[1,6] Therefore, when depression subsides, it is considered to be in remission instead of cured, as symptoms are managed but may recur in the future. It is important for youth to understand some key symptoms of depression and potential stress triggers to help mitigate future impact and for them to engage in early intervention to help offset additional full depressive episodes. If multiple depressive episodes (chronic) have occurred, clinicians should consider keeping maintenance strategies (eg, therapy and medication) active even though patients feel better and can participate in their daily routine.

➤ What is the process to wean a patient off an SSRI?

Treatment: Depression Remission

In general, SSRIs are weaned slowly over months and are tapered not in standard increments (ie, 25 mg) but rather as a proportion of the previous dose (ie, 25%).[34]

How quickly one tapers depends partly on how long they have been taking the medication and how high their dose currently is. In this case, Savannah has been taking her medication for 1 year and is at a mid-therapeutic dose, so a tapering plan of 50% every 4 weeks would be appropriate.

The following example taper regimen shows the number of weeks and the corresponding dosage for Savannah:

- Current dose: 15 mg
- First taper: 10 mg for 4 weeks
- Second taper: 5 mg for 4 weeks
- Third taper: 2.5 mg for 4 weeks

During a medication taper, close follow-up is recommended to monitor for both adverse effects and symptom recurrence. If adolescents become impatient and taper more quickly than recommended or stop taking their medication, they may experience discontinuation symptoms (refer to Chapter 11, Depression and Depressive Disorder, for more information). While the patient is tapering, validated screening tools should be used to trend scores and compare them with prior results.

Back to the Case: Depression Recurrence or New Diagnosis

Savannah has now been off her escitalopram for 4 months and is seeing you for her annual health supervision visit with her parents. Her PHQ-A score is 0, but in the office, you note her affect to be flat. She reports that she's always fighting with her mom and that she hasn't been feeling well. Her mom agrees that her mood is irritable most days at mom's house, but her dad says she is just a normal teenager and they find ways to have fun together. Dad's only concern is that she still has trouble sleeping at night and can't fall asleep unless he gives her melatonin. You note on her growth chart that although she has always had a weight at the fifth percentile, she is now dropping off the growth chart, with a 10-lb weight loss over the past 2 months. When you discuss this, she says, "I've always been small, so I don't see why you are making a big deal of it now. I don't want to be fat."

Differential Diagnosis: Depression Recurrence or New Diagnosis

In this case, there is a known history of depression, but whether her new mood changes and weight loss are related to a depression recurrence or a new diagnosis needs to be considered. The differential diagnosis of weight loss is vast, so the clinician will need to think broadly and then narrow down according to the evaluation.

- **Depression recurrence:** Her normal PHQ-A score is reassuring, but there is a notable flat affect in the office, irritable mood at her mom's house, and ongoing issues with sleep.
- **Endocrine disorder**
  - Thyroid disease
  - Addison disease
- **Gastrointestinal disorder**
  - Celiac disease
  - Irritable bowel syndrome
  - Inflammatory bowel disease (IBD)
  - Superior mesenteric artery syndrome
  - Wilson disease
- **Vitamin D deficiency**
- **Malignancy**
- **Infection**
  - HIV infection
  - Epstein-Barr virus infection
  - Tuberculosis
  - Syphilis
- **Eating disorder**
  - Anorexia nervosa
  - Bulimia nervosa

Evaluation: Depression Recurrence or New Diagnosis

If unsure about the validity of her PHQ-A score, the clinician could consider screening for depression recurrence by using another validated tool, such as the Pediatric Symptom Checklist-17 (PSC-17). In addition, the AAP recommends universally screening youth 12 years and older for suicide, and the ASQ is a 4-item screening tool used for children as young as 8 years, with a high sensitivity and specificity for detecting suicide risk.[4–6,35] In one study, 32% of children with suicidal ideation who were missed by the PHQ-A were identified by the ASQ.[5] If the ASQ is positive, this should be followed by a brief suicide assessment tool like the C-SSRS. Refer to the Appendix for links to the tools online.

To further narrow down the differential diagnosis, consider the following laboratory evaluation:

- Complete blood cell count
- Ferritin level
- Comprehensive metabolic panel with magnesium and phosphorus levels
- Thyrotropin (previously referred to as *thyroid-stimulating hormone*) with reflex to free thyroxine function
- Celiac disease panel

- Erythrocyte sedimentation rate and C-reactive protein level
- 25-Hydroxyvitamin D
- Amylase and lipase levels

Depending on further history (including sexual history, travel history, and exposures), the clinician may add

- HIV screening
- Epstein-Barr virus serology
- Quantiferon-TB Gold Plus or purified protein derivative test
- Rapid plasma reagin test

If there is a concern for disordered eating, check orthostatic vital signs and ask about menstrual history to assess for amenorrhea. Additionally, scheduling an electrocardiogram (ECG) may be useful.

Inpatient admission for medical care is indicated if any of the following findings are present[36–39]:

- Physiological instability
- Bradycardia (<50 beats per minute [bpm])
- Hypotension (<90/45 mm Hg)
- Hypothermia (<96° F)
- Orthostatic changes (>40 bpm pulse change or >20 mm Hg systolic or >10 mm Hg diastolic blood pressure change)
- Acute medical complications of malnutrition, such as syncope
- Abnormal ECG findings
- Less than 75% of a median body mass index (%mBMI)
- Abnormal serum electrolyte levels, including
  - Potassium less than 3.2 mmol/L
  - Chloride less than 88 mmol/L
  - Phosphorus less than 3.0 mg/dL
  - Sodium less than 132 mmol/L

Other considerations that may warrant inpatient admission are[38]

- Arrested growth and development
- Failure of outpatient treatment
- Acute food refusal
- Uncontrollable binge eating and purging
- Coexisting psychiatric or medical condition that prohibits or limits outpatient treatment

A helpful clinical pathway for the inpatient evaluation and treatment of children with weight loss, malnutrition, and eating disorders can be found online (www.chop.edu/clinical-pathway/malnutrition-weight-loss-eating-disorders-clinical-pathway).

In this case, Savannah does not have any laboratory markers for inpatient admission but does seem to have an eating disorder (based on the following diagnostic criteria for anorexia nervosa)[40]:

- Low body weight caused by restrictive intake
- Fear of gaining weight
- Persistent lack of recognition of the seriousness of current low body weight[38,40]

Given that the patient has a history of anxiety and now has weight loss, interference with psychosocial functioning, and no concurrent medical condition to explain her weight loss, is there a reason to suspect avoidant/restrictive food intake disorder (ARFID) rather than anorexia nervosa?

Avoidant/restrictive food intake disorder is associated with weight loss, significant nutritional deficiency, dependence on nutritional supplementation, and/or marked interference with psychosocial functioning.[40] However, unlike with anorexia nervosa, there is no disturbance in how one perceives their own body.[36,39,40] In many cases, ARFID presents with food avoidance or restriction based on a sensory experience with food or eating. Sometimes these patients have a history of being called "picky eaters" and may have had a feeding disorder of infancy or early childhood.[36,39] In other cases, these individuals may start avoiding foods after an adverse experience, such as choking, anaphylaxis, or repeated vomiting caused by illness.[36,38]

In this case, Savannah demonstrates a fear of gaining weight ("I don't want to be fat"), a disturbance in how she perceives her own body ("I've always been small"), and lack of recognition of the seriousness of current low body weight ("I don't see why you are making a big deal"), which are not features of ARFID. Refer to the *Diagnostic and Statistical Manual of Mental Disorders, Fifth Edition, Text Revision* for full diagnostic criteria.[40]

Savannah's family asks if her disordered eating was triggered by weaning off the escitalopram.

The etiology of disordered eating is multifactorial and includes biological, psychological, environmental, and sociocultural factors.[36,38,39]

Children or adolescents at increased risk for disordered eating include those with[37,39–41]

- A history of anxiety, obsessive-compulsive disorder (OCD), autism spectrum disorder, childhood obesity, or preterm birth
- A family history of eating disorders
- A sexual minority identity
- Chronic health conditions (eg, diabetes, celiac disease, IBD)
- Restrictive dieting (eg, veganism, orthorexia nervosa)
- Bullying history

- Sexual abuse history
- Avocations that encourage thinness (eg, modeling, elite athletics)

Coexisting psychiatric disorders are common with disordered eating, including anxiety, OCD, substance use disorder, autism, and attention-deficit/hyperactivity disorder.[36,38,39] Having a coexisting psychiatric disorder tends to worsen the prognosis of an eating disorder because it may interfere with the treatment plan, and symptoms can be overlapping. Suicidal ideation and behaviors are also increased in patients with eating disorders, and death by suicide is 18 times more likely in patients with anorexia nervosa.[32,38]

No medications are approved by the FDA for the treatment of anorexia nervosa. Fluoxetine has been approved by the FDA for the treatment of bulimia nervosa. When SSRIs are used in patients with disordered eating, they are to treat coexisting diagnoses, such as anxiety or depression.[38]

Because there is no evidence that SSRIs treat disordered eating, the weaning off of Savannah's escitalopram in this case did not unmask her eating disorder and is coincidental to the development. Ongoing close screening and assessment for anxiety and depression is indicated, especially in the context of her having prior diagnoses of both. In addition, ongoing screening and assessment for suicidality is important.

Keep in Mind: Caring for Oneself

Burnout, secondary traumatic stress, and compassion fatigue can all be experienced by health care professionals who care for pediatric patients with mental health concerns. If a clinician is experiencing any of these symptoms, they should try to

- Connect with their emotions through mindfulness, self-reflection, or journaling.
- Seek professional support from a mental health specialist.
- Maintain healthy boundaries between themselves and their work/patients.
- Practice self-compassion by avoiding negative self-talk and being kind to themselves.

Management: Disordered Eating

Collaborative management between a multidisciplinary team, which may include the clinician, nurses, nutritionists, and mental health specialists, is important. The pediatric clinician should serve as the coordinator of referrals and the person who ensures that the patient receives the right level of care. Management of disordered eating in the office setting includes[36,38,39]

- Family-based therapy: the gold standard approach to eating disorder treatment, to be recommended above other individual-based therapy options if possible[37,39,42]
  - Other therapy options
    - Enhanced cognitive behavioral therapy
    - Dialectical behavior therapy
    - Acceptance and commitment therapy
    - Wraparound services/in-home services
- Close supervision of meals by parents/caregivers, as instructed by a mental health specialist or nutritionist[39]
  - The patient should eat 3 meals and 2 to 3 snacks each day.
  - Meals should include a variety of foods (meat, starch, dairy, fruits, vegetables, and fats).
  - Foods marketed as "diet foods" should be avoided.
- Promotion of food neutrality and avoidance of labeling foods as "good," "bad," "junk," or "healthy"; encouragement of the patient and family to think of food as medicine
- Weighing the patient in a gown only with the weight hidden from the patient at checks in the pediatric office until the patient becomes established with a disordered eating treatment program or specialized multidisciplinary treatment team

Weight restoration is an important goal of early treatment, but determining the degree of malnutrition present requires standardized classification. The AAP and Society for Adolescent Health and Medicine recommend using %mBMI, BMI z scores, and amount and rate of weight loss to classify a patient with mild, moderate, or severe malnutrition.[37,39] Treatment goal weight (TGW) is the weight necessary to support healthy growth and development, and calculation of TGW should consider the youth's prior trajectory for height, weight, and BMI; age at pubertal onset; current sexual maturity rating; and parental heights.[37,39] Treatment goal weight may be calculated with the help of a nutritionist with experience with eating disorders and often needs to be recalculated every 3 to 6 months.

Close and frequent observation is warranted for outpatient treatment failure that would prompt referral to a day treatment program or inpatient treatment program.

Conclusion

In this case, the complexity of managing the care for a patient with coexisting mental health diagnoses is seen. Frequent screening for recurrence, as well as new diagnoses, is important throughout the evaluation and management for a patient. Positive results on a screening tool, such as one for suicidal ideation, should be followed by thorough assessment of the patient. The pediatric clinician serves a critical role in early detection and in facilitation of appropriate referrals to higher levels of care, mental health specialists, or inpatient/outpatient treatment facilities.

Lessons Learned From the Snowball

A strengths-based approach is important in the Snowball case (as suicidality and eating disorder unfold), as these patients are prone to sad mood, withdrawn behavior, and negative self-talk. Suicide screening should occur universally and throughout the management period. Close monitoring for coexisting conditions can help with early identification and improve the chances of patients being able to manage symptoms as an outpatient and improve prognosis. Additionally, these patients should always place a priority on daily wellness factors, such as proper sleep hygiene, social connections, and a focus on proper nutrition and physical activity.

- Suicidal ideation can occur at any point during depression management and should be screened for universally.[5,6]
- Selective serotonin reuptake inhibitors contain a black box warning about increased suicidal thoughts, but not acts, particularly at the time of initiation and dose titration.[17]
- A positive suicide screening result needs to be followed by an assessment, which includes exploration for a method, plan, and intent, as well as protective factors and safety planning.[7]
- Safety planning includes helping a patient recognize warning signs, identify internal and external coping strategies, identify contacts and distractions, learn how to ask for help, and identify professional crisis resources.[19]
- Disordered eating and suicidal ideation are often coexisting.[38,39]
- Disordered eating management should be multidisciplinary, including team members such as a pediatric clinician, nutritionist, and mental health specialist.
- Nutritional rehabilitation, medical stability, and family-based therapy are the mainstays of anorexia nervosa treatment, and psychopharmacology is not indicated (unless treating an active coexisting mental health diagnosis).[38,39]

Keywords: anorexia nervosa, ARFID, disordered eating, eating disorder, safety planning, suicidal ideation, suicidality, suicide, 988

Suggested Reading

Acosta W, Qayyum Z, Turban JL, van Schalkwyk GI. Identify, engage, understand: supporting transgender youth in an inpatient psychiatric hospital. *Psychiatr Q.* 2019;90(3):601–612 PMID: 31209713

March JS, Silva S, Petrycki S, et al. The Treatment for Adolescents With Depression Study (TADS): long-term effectiveness and safety outcomes. *Arch Gen Psychiatry.* 2007;64(10):1132–1143 PMID: 17909125

Rodan SC, Bryant E, Le A, et al; National Eating Disorder Research Consortium. Pharmacotherapy, alternative and adjunctive therapies for eating disorders: findings from a rapid review. *J Eat Disord.* 2023;11(1):112 PMID: 37415200

Soffer S, Lewis J, Marroquin Y. Outpatient clinical pathway for assessment and care planning for children and adolescents at risk for suicide. Children's Hospital of Philadelphia. June 2019. Updated November 2025. Accessed February 12, 2026. https://www.chop.edu/clinical-pathway/suicide-risk-assessment-and-care-planning-clinical-pathway

Weersing VR, Jeffreys M, Do MT, Schwartz KTG, Bolano C. Evidence base update of psychosocial treatments for child and adolescent depression. *J Clin Child Adolesc Psychol.* 2017;46(1):11–43 PMID: 27870579

References

1. American Psychiatric Association. Depressive disorders. In: *Diagnostic and Statistical Manual of Mental Disorders.* 5th ed, text rev. American Psychiatric Association Publishing; 2022:177–214
2. Posner K, Brown GK, Stanley B, et al. The Columbia-Suicide Severity Rating Scale: initial validity and internal consistency findings from three multisite studies with adolescents and adults. *Am J Psychiatry.* 2011;168(12):1266–1277 PMID: 22193671
3. Research Foundation for Mental Hygiene Inc. The Columbia Lighthouse Project. Accessed February 12, 2026. https://cssrs.columbia.edu
4. Horowitz LM, Bridge JA, Teach SJ, et al. Ask Suicide-Screening Questions (ASQ): a brief instrument for the pediatric emergency department. *Arch Pediatr Adolesc Med.* 2012;166(12):1170–1176 PMID: 23027429
5. Horowitz LM, Mournet AM, Lanzillo E, et al. Screening pediatric medical patients for suicide risk: is depression screening enough? *J Adolesc Health.* 2021;68(6):1183–1188 PMID: 33712380
6. Zuckerbrot RA, Cheung A, Jensen PS, Stein REK, Laraque D; GLAD-PC Steering Group. Guidelines for Adolescent Depression in Primary Care (GLAD-PC), I: practice preparation, identification, assessment, and initial management. *Pediatrics.* 2018;141(3):e20174081 PMID: 29483200
7. Pettit JW, Buitron V, Green KL. Assessment and management of suicide risk in children and adolescents. *Cogn Behav Pract.* 2018;25(4):460–472 PMID: 31787833
8. Miranda-Mendizabal A, Castellví P, Parés-Badell O, et al. Gender differences in suicidal behavior in adolescents and young adults: systematic review and meta-analysis of longitudinal studies. *Int J Public Health.* 2019;64(2):265–283 PMID: 30635683
9. Nock MK, Borges G, Bromet EJ, et al. Cross-national prevalence and risk factors for suicidal ideation, plans and attempts. *Br J Psychiatry.* 2008;192(2):98–105 PMID: 18245022
10. Prades-Caballero V, Navarro-Pérez JJ, Carbonell Á. factors associated with suicidal behavior in adolescents: an umbrella review using the socio-ecological model. *Community Ment Health J.* 2025;61(4):612–628 PMID: 39487937

11. Shatkin JP. *Child & Adolescent Mental Health: A Practical, All-in-One Guide.* 3rd ed. WW Norton & Co; 2024:258–259
12. The Trevor Project. 2022 National Survey on LGBTQ Youth Mental Health. Accessed February 12, 2026. https://www.thetrevorproject.org/survey-2022
13. Seager van Dyk I, Sena R, McCord C, Kodish T, DeAntonio M. Affirming LGBTQIA+ youth in inpatient psychiatric settings. *J Am Acad Child Adolesc Psychiatry.* 2024;63(3):296–300 PMID: 37451313
14. O'Halloran L, Coey P, Wilson C. Suicidality in autistic youth: a systematic review and meta-analysis. *Clin Psychol Rev.* 2022;93:102144 PMID: 35290800
15. Meyer IH. Prejudice, social stress, and mental health in lesbian, gay, and bisexual populations: conceptual issues and research evidence. *Psychol Bull.* 2003;129(5):674–697 PMID: 12956539
16. Akkas F. Youth suicide risk increased over past decade: new national data highlights concerning trends among high schoolers. Pew Charitable Trusts. March 3, 2023. Updated March 7, 2023. Accessed February 12, 2026. https://www.pew.org/en/research-and-analysis/articles/2023/03/03/youth-suicide-risk-increased-over-past-decade
17. US Food and Drug Administration. Suicidality in children and adolescents being treated with antidepressant medications. February 5, 2018. Accessed February 12, 2026. https://www.fda.gov/drugs/postmarket-drug-safety-information-patients-and-providers/suicidality-children-and-adolescents-being-treated-antidepressant-medications
18. Cheung AH, Zuckerbrot RA, Jensen PS, et al. GLAD-PC Steering Group. Guidelines for Adolescent Depression in Primary Care (GLAD-PC), II: treatment and ongoing management. *Pediatrics.* 2018;141(3):e20174082 PMID: 29483201
19. Stanley B, Brown GK. Safety planning intervention: a brief intervention to mitigate suicide risk. *Cogn Behav Pract.* 2012;19(2):256–264
20. Lee LK, Fleegler EW, Goyal MK, et al; American Academy of Pediatrics Council on Injury, Violence, and Poison Prevention. Firearm-related injuries and deaths in children and youth: injury prevention and harm reduction. *Pediatrics.* 2022;150(6):e2022060070 PMID: 36207776
21. Sobanski T, Josfeld S, Peikert G, Wagner G. Psychotherapeutic interventions for the prevention of suicide re-attempts: a systematic review. *Psychol Med.* 2021;51(15):2525–2540 PMID: 34608856
22. Gomez K, Canon T, Barr EA. Cognitive-behavioral therapy and suicide risk in adolescents and young adults: a systematic review. *J Psychosoc Nurs Ment Health Serv.* 2025;63(8):14–23 PMID: 40067194
23. Asarnow JR, Hughes JL, Babeva KN, Sugar CA. Cognitive-behavioral family treatment for suicide attempt prevention: a randomized controlled trial. *J Am Acad Child Adolesc Psychiatry.* 2017;56(6):506–514 PMID: 28545756
24. Büscher R, Torok M, Terhorst Y, Sander L. Internet-based cognitive behavioral therapy to reduce suicidal ideation: a systematic review and meta-analysis. *JAMA Netw Open.* 2020;3(4):e203933 PMID: 32343354
25. Sander LB, Beisemann M, Doebler P, et al. The effects of internet-based cognitive behavioral therapy for suicidal ideation or behaviors on depression, anxiety, and hopelessness in individuals with suicidal ideation: systematic review and meta-analysis of individual participant data. *J Med Internet Res.* 2023;25:e46771 PMID: 37358893
26. McCauley E, Berk MS, Asarnow JR, et al. Efficacy of dialectical behavior therapy for adolescents at high risk for suicide: a randomized clinical trial. *JAMA Psychiatry.* 2018;75(8):777–785 PMID: 29926087
27. Kothgassner OD, Goreis A, Robinson K, Huscsava MM, Schmahl C, Plener PL. Efficacy of dialectical behavior therapy for adolescent self-harm and suicidal ideation: a systematic review and meta-analysis. *Psychol Med.* 2021;51(7):1057–1067 PMID: 33875025

28. Sullivan SR, Myhre K, Mitchell EL, et al. Suicide and telehealth treatments: A PRISMA scoping review. *Arch Suicide Res*. 2022;26(4):1794–1814 PMID: 35137677
29. Baker JC, Starkey A, Ammendola E, et al. Telehealth brief cognitive behavioral therapy for suicide prevention: a randomized clinical trial. *JAMA Netw Open*. 2024;7(11):e2445913 PMID: 39531231
30. Hamza CA, Willoughby T. Nonsuicidal self-injury and suicidal risk among emerging adults. *J Adolesc Health*. 2016;59(4):411–415 PMID: 27485906
31. Whitlock J, Muehlenkamp J, Eckenrode J, et al. Nonsuicidal self-injury as a gateway to suicide in young adults. *J Adolesc Health*. 2013;52(4):486–492 PMID: 23298982
32. Glenn CR, Franklin JC, Nock MK. Evidence-based psychosocial treatments for self-injurious thoughts and behaviors in youth. *J Clin Child Adolesc Psychol*. 2015;44(1):1–29 PMID: 25256034
33. Chung RJ, Lee JB, Hackell JM, Alderman EM; American Academy of Pediatrics Committee on Adolescence and Committee on Practice and Ambulatory Medicine. Confidentiality in the care of adolescents: policy statement. *Pediatrics*. 2024;153(5):e2024066326 PMID: 38646690
34. Horowitz MA, Taylor D. Tapering of SSRI treatment to mitigate withdrawal symptoms. *Lancet Psychiatry*. 2019;6(6):538–546 PMID: 30850328
35. Saidinejad M, Duffy S, Wallin D, et al; American Academy of Pediatrics Committee on Pediatric Emergency Medicine; American College of Emergency Physicians Pediatric Emergency Medicine Committee; Emergency Nurses Association Pediatric Committee. The management of children and youth with pediatric mental and behavioral health emergencies. *Pediatrics*. 2023;152(3):e2023063256 PMID: 37584106
36. Noonan EM, Solfermoser B, Heller K. Eating disorders. *Pediatr Rev*. 2025;46(6):291–303 PMID: 40449905
37. Golden NH, Katzman DK, Rome ES, et al; Society for Adolescent Health and Medicine. Medical management of restrictive eating disorders in adolescents and young adults. *J Adolesc Health*. 2022;71(5):648–654 PMID: 36058805
38. Frostad S, Bentz M. Anorexia nervosa: outpatient treatment and medical management. *World J Psychiatry*. 2022;12(4):558–579 PMID: 35582333
39. Hornberger LL, Lane MA; American Academy of Pediatrics Committee on Adolescence. Identification and management of eating disorders in children and adolescents. *Pediatrics*. 2021;147(1):e2020040279 PMID: 33386343
40. American Psychiatric Association. Feeding and eating disorders. In: *Diagnostic and Statistical Manual of Mental Disorders*. 5th ed, text rev. American Psychiatric Association Publishing; 2022:371–397
41. Schneider M. Eating abnormalities. In: Foy JM, ed. *Mental Health Care of Children and Adolescents: A Guide for Primary Care Clinicians*. American Academy of Pediatrics; 2018
42. Forsberg S, Lock J. Family-based treatment of child and adolescent eating disorders. *Child Adolesc Psychiatr Clin N Am*. 2015;24(3):617–629 PMID: 26092743

Part 2

Symptom Management and Initial Treatment

CHAPTER 10

Anxiety and Anxiety Disorder

Treatment of patients with subthreshold anxiety symptoms or anxiety disorders can be initiated in the pediatric primary care setting. The American Academy of Pediatrics (AAP) endorses that in order to promote the optimal development of children, behavioral and emotional screening should happen routinely in pediatric primary care so early intervention can occur. Pediatric clinicians are well positioned to address the behavioral and mental health of their patients because of their longitudinal relationships with patients and their families, whole-child approach, and ability to initiate treatment and/or serve as a bridge to mental health specialists.[1,2]

Screening for anxiety and assessment of impairment were discussed in the cases in Chapters 1, Somatic Symptoms or Panic Disorder; 2, Separation Anxiety; and 3, Perfectionism. Some cases presented subthreshold anxiety symptoms that caused impairment in functioning but did not rise to the level of a clinical diagnosis, while others met criteria for a disorder and required a higher level of clinical and medical intervention. It is important to understand the difference between the two to find the best avenue for care and management in the clinical setting. Anxiety in and of itself should not be pathologized, as it can serve a vital and important role in survival and daily living; thus, helping patients distinguish between managing symptoms and managing a disorder is an important distinction. While diagnostic criteria for anxiety disorders will be reviewed, the purpose of this chapter is to review psychoeducation, psychotherapy, medication management, referral to psychologists or psychiatrists, and the comanagement of patients with anxiety.

As a reminder, screening tools should not be used to provide a diagnosis alone. Screening tools are brief and standardized, as a way to better understand impairing symptoms and flag individuals who may be at risk of developing a disorder. If the results from a screening tool warrant further evaluation, the patient should be referred to a mental health specialist for a full workup, which will include components such as validated assessment instruments and clinical interviews, administered by trained professionals, to determine if diagnostic criteria are met. When discussing treatment options for anxiety with a patient, it is important to provide the patient with psychoeducation about anxiety, including its impact on functioning; evidence-based treatment options; medication options (if applicable); and brief interventions to help maintain and stabilize the patient's mood and functioning in one's role as the primary care clinician.

Keep in Mind: A Primary Care Clinician's Role

- Facilitate brief interventions in the office setting, including evidence-based screening tools.
- Initiate first-line medications as clinically indicated.
- Provide referrals to mental health specialists.
- Provide supportive monitoring until a mental health specialist is involved and the patient's condition is stable with medication.

Review the Diagnostic Criteria for Anxiety Disorders

In a perfect world, a clinician would be able to use a brief screening tool and then refer a patient for follow-up intervention if a diagnostic evaluation were warranted. However, because of pediatric mental health specialist shortages or extended wait times for appointments, pediatric primary care clinicians often need to manage their patient's mental health care issues.[3–5] Therefore, it is important for these clinicians to understand how to assess for conditions like anxiety disorders. As always, seek consultation and team-based collaboration with mental health specialists whenever possible.

To assess for anxiety issues and potential anxiety disorders, use a clinical interview (eg, with patient and multiple raters such as parents/caregivers and schools/teachers); criteria from the *Diagnostic and Statistical Manual of Mental Disorders, Fifth Edition, Text Revision;* and brief, standardized screening tools (eg, Screen for Child Anxiety Related Emotional Disorders [SCARED], Generalized Anxiety Disorder-7 [GAD-7], Pediatric Symptom Checklist-17 [PSC-17]), in addition to assessment of functional impairment to make a preliminary diagnosis of anxiety disorder. Refer to the Appendix for descriptions and links to the tools online. Typical anxiety disorder diagnoses in pediatric primary care include

- **Generalized anxiety disorder (GAD)[6]:** characterized by an intense and uncontrollable worry (for at least 6 months) about a variety of potential problems; typically, not something that the individual needs to worry about (eg, school performance, personal or caregiver safety, future events or performance)
- **Social anxiety disorder[7]:** characterized by intense fear in or about social settings beyond shyness or slowness to warm; avoidance of social interactions; fear of peer rejection; and somatic symptoms, such as headaches, muscular tension, restlessness, and palpitations, that appear to improve when the individual is avoiding social interactions

- **Separation anxiety disorder[8]:** characterized by intense fear of being separated from a caregiver beyond what is typically expected; fear of either personal safety or caregiver safety when the individual and caregiver are apart; and tearfulness and somatic complaints
- **Panic disorder[9]:** characterized by intense somatic feelings in the body (eg, rapid heartbeat, rapid breathing, dizziness, sweating, nausea, chest pain); maladaptive cognitions (eg, "I think I'm having a heart attack"); and avoidance of people, places, or situations that might induce panic behavior

A patient must have symptoms for 4 or more weeks for separation anxiety and panic disorder and 6 or more months for generalized anxiety and social anxiety disorder. In addition, the diagnosis of anxiety is made when there is significant impairment or distress from the anxiety symptoms.

Psychoeducation

Everyone has emotions, and all feelings are normal. Anxiety exists in everyone, and at low levels, it can help people feel motivated to stay away from danger or think through their actions at times. However, it is a person's reaction, and sometimes their overreaction, to those emotions that can create challenges and interfere with daily functioning. Sharing this information with a patient or family can help normalize some of the fears they have. With anxiety, typically the reaction to the stressor is avoidance of it, or the cessation or withdrawal from an activity or action because the fear or worry is too intense and causes stress or somatic symptoms. When these reactions interfere with functioning, the next step may be to consider treatment of the anxiety. Treatment should help patients identify triggers such as negative thoughts or excessive worries, help change maladaptive thoughts to more helpful ones, and provide therapeutic exercises to turn these more helpful thoughts into actions or prosocial behaviors (through exposures). Build a therapeutic alliance with the patient and family by displaying empathy, normalizing feelings, and empowering patients to speak about their feelings. The HEL^2P^3 mnemonic, developed by the AAP Task Force on Mental Health, can be used to build trust and develop a plan of care.[4]

- H = Hope.
- E = Empathy.
- L^2 = Language, Loyalty.
- P^3 = Permission, Partnership, Plan.

Evidence-Based Treatment Options

The Child/Adolescent Anxiety Multimodal Study (CAMS) was a treatment-focused randomized controlled trial of youth with moderate to severe anxiety disorders.[10] Participants were randomized to a placebo arm or 1 of 3 treatment groups, including sertraline alone, cognitive behavioral therapy (CBT) alone, or a combination of sertraline and CBT (Box 10-1).

Box 10-1. Improvement Rates by Treatment Groups and Placebo Arm in the Child/Adolescent Anxiety Multimodal Study[a]

- 81% combination (CBT and medication)
- 60% CBT only
- 55% medication only
- 24% placebo

Abbreviation: CBT, cognitive behavioral therapy.

[a] Compton SN, Walkup JT, Albano AM, et al. Child/Adolescent Anxiety Multimodal Study (CAMS): rationale, design, and methods. *Child Adolesc Psychiatry Ment Health.* 2010;4:1.

At 12 weeks, all treatment groups fared superior to the placebo arm, and the combination of sertraline and CBT was significantly more effective than sertraline or CBT alone.[10] However, as the 3 treatment groups were followed up over time, the rates of efficacy became comparable and set forth guidelines for when which type of treatment is the most efficacious (Box 10-2).[10] This study helped determine that a combination approach of psychotherapy and psychopharmacology is recommended in the initial treatment of moderate to severe anxiety.

Box 10-2. Anxiety Management by Severity[a]

- **Mild:** psychotherapy alone
- **Moderate:** psychotherapy + consideration of pharmacotherapy
- **Severe:** psychotherapy + pharmacotherapy

[a] Compton SN, Walkup JT, Albano AM, et al. Child/Adolescent Anxiety Multimodal Study (CAMS): rationale, design, and methods. *Child Adolesc Psychiatry Ment Health.* 2010;4:1.

Psychotherapy

Cognitive behavioral therapy is the psychotherapy program with the most evidence for the treatment of anxiety.[11,12] It focuses on identifying and challenging negative thought patterns and their resulting behaviors, and it highlights the way that feelings, behaviors, and thoughts are interconnected (Figure 10–1). Psychoeducation, gradual exposures, somatic management skills training, cognitive strategies such as cognitive restructuring tasks, parental support, and relapse prevention plans are all parts of CBT.[11,12] It is present focused and problem-solving oriented to address real-time interference with functioning and reduce avoidance.[11]

Figure 10-1. Components of Cognitive Behavioral Therapy

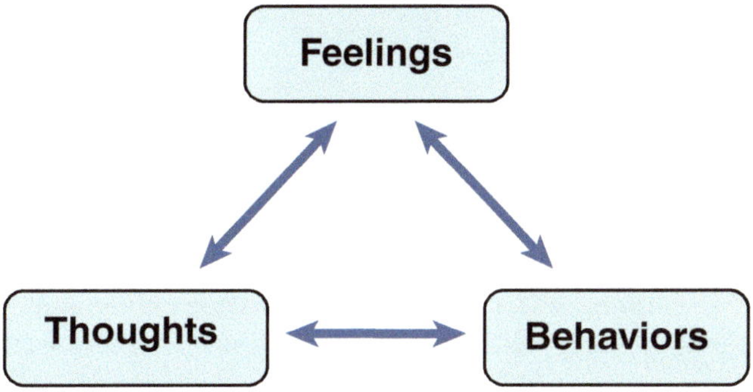

Keep in Mind: Therapy Recommendations

Because not all therapists use CBT in their approach to treating anxiety, when providing a recommendation for therapy, the clinician should refer to CBT by name and suggest that families ask for and seek out this specific type of evidence-based therapy.

If a patient's anxiety is the result of a traumatic incident, consider referring them for trauma-focused cognitive behavioral therapy (TF-CBT), which uses the same components of CBT with a trauma-focused lens to address the symptoms of trauma and posttraumatic stress. It can be helpful for co-occurring depression, anxiety, and other behavioral issues stemming from trauma.

When the patient is in established CBT therapy, the clinician can ask about what types of things they have learned and actions they have performed, such as

- **Gradual exposures** (eg, slowly exposing themselves to things they fear, such as insects or public speaking, in a careful and planned manner)

- **Cognitive restructuring tasks** (eg, changing unhelpful thoughts to helpful ones, such as "Even though tests are scary for me, I tend to do well and get high grades")
- **Somatic management skills training** (eg, deep breathing or relaxation training to help with stomachaches or racing heartbeats)[12]

Include caregivers in the conversation by asking what they have learned to help support change in their children. Sometimes the clinician can use a rating scale to help get a subjective opinion on treatment progress (eg, "When I saw you last time for your social anxiety, you rated the stressful feelings as 9/10, with 10 as the worst imaginable anxious feelings. Now, as you are in therapy, how would you rate that stressful thought?"). Opening a dialogue such as this can help with progress monitoring.

Additional Therapies

There are other therapies that could be beneficial in improving functioning once CBT has been established (concurrent) or completed. These types of therapies can include, but are not limited to, family therapy (especially when anxiety is a family-dominant trait that affects many in the household), dialectical behavior therapy and skills group (for teens, particularly those with issues in executive functioning),[13] play therapy (for younger children), psychodynamic therapy, and exposure and response prevention for obsessive-compulsive disorder (OCD).

Brief Interventions and Continuity of Care

It is important to maintain a connection with patients and their families while they seek treatment or wait for an appointment. The clinician can suggest quick, active, and simple strategies that can help address the cognitive and somatic impairments of anxiety. Consider promoting strategies that involve healthy habits, relaxation and mindfulness, and careful reclamation of negative thoughts.[11,14–16]

Lifestyle Modifications

- Focus on improving sleep hygiene; make sure the child is falling asleep at a reasonable hour and getting adequate nighttime sleep.
- Limit screen time to help increase physical activity, promote social/family interaction, and inhibit impact on sleep hygiene.[17,18]
- Reduce caffeine consumption or other self-medicating strategies (eg, alcohol to ease social anxiety feelings).
- Increase physical activity.
- Limit/monitor social media use. Research has shown that greater social media use is significantly associated with internalizing problems, including anxiety and depression.[19–21]

Relaxation and Mindfulness

- Place large emphasis on the importance of deep breathing and relaxation techniques.
  - For younger children
    - Flower breathing: Pretend to hold a flower in your hand. Now slowly breathe in all the pretty smell of the flower. Now slowly try to blow the petals off one by one. Repeat this with a different-color flower.
    - Birthday candle breathing: Imagine you have a birthday cake with 4 candles on it and you need to blow them out. Slowly take a deep breath in through your nose, then very slowly blow the candles out one by one (to the count of 4) until all the air is out. Now try it with 5 candles.
  - For older children/teens
    - 5-finger breathing: Hold up one hand, and with the other, trace your fingers. As you trace up, inhale, and as you trace down, exhale. Repeat this 3 times.
    - Box breathing: Trace an imaginary box with your finger in the air, each side taking 4 seconds. Breathe in (4 seconds), hold your breath (4 seconds), exhale (4 seconds), and hold your breath (4 seconds). Repeat this 3 times.
- Mindfulness and grounding
    - Grounding technique: Name 5 things you can see, 4 things you can touch, 3 things you can hear, 2 things you can smell, and 1 thing you can taste.
    - Affirmations: Choose an empowering phrase with short phrases that you can tap out on your fingers. For example, "I am in control" or "I will be OK."

Keep in Mind: Incorporating Mindfulness Techniques Into Examinations

- Demonstrate box breathing with a patient during the respiratory examination. While tracing the box, they are silent, so with each inhale/exhale, their breath sounds should be clearly heard.
- Identify an affirmation or a reclamation for a patient who feels anxious about vaccines to use before and during vaccine administrations (eg, a 4-syllable affirmation such as "I can do this" or a reclamation of negative thoughts such as "This may hurt, but it will be over so fast, so I can be brave"). Have them practice these techniques before and during their vaccine administrations.

Cognitive Restructuring and Overactive Worry

- Addressing negative thoughts: Red light/green light game—First describe how a traffic light works (ie, red light = stop; green light = go). Then explain that a negative thought is a "red thought" and help the patient identify a red thought they may have, such as "I'm terrible at tests and going to fail." The point of the game is to change a red thought to a "green thought" when it occurs. So instead of "I'm going to fail," the patient changes it to a green thought, such as "I typically do well on tests" or "I studied, so I will try my best."
- Creating structured "worry time": Have the patient set aside 15 minutes a day for worry time. During this time, they sit with a parent or caregiver and discuss all their worries. When worry time is up, they move on with the day. If worries come up throughout the next day, they write them down so they will remember them at the next worry time. Worry time can be at any time except before bedtime.

For patients who are being referred to a mental health specialist, the strategies described in this section can be initiated to offer them some tools to address symptoms of anxiety while they await therapy. These strategies are equally useful for symptoms that present during stressful patient care encounters. Educate patients and families about other resources, such as apps, books/workbooks, or websites, that they can use to build skills and feel more confident in managing anxiety symptoms at home. Many of these resources use some of the same approaches and techniques that patients will learn in psychotherapy and can be a helpful bridge for improving daily functioning until they establish care with their mental health specialist.

Resources

Apps

We expect technology to change over time and encourage readers to find apps endorsed by groups such as the American Academy of Pediatrics, the American Psychological Association, and the American Academy of Child and Adolescent Psychiatry. Clinicians can work with families to identify apps that may be helpful for their specific needs.

Books for Parents and Caregivers

- *Helping Your Anxious Child: A Step-by-Step Guide*, 3rd Edition, by Ronald Rapee, PhD; Ann Wignall, DPsych; Susan Spence, PhD; Vanessa Cobham, PhD; and Heidi Lyneham, PhD

Books/Workbooks for Children

- *Anxiety Relief for Kids: On-the-Spot Strategies to Help Your Child Overcome Worry, Panic, and Avoidance* by Bridge Flynn Walker, PhD
- *What to Do When Mistakes Make You Quake: A Kid's Guide to Accepting Imperfection*, Revised Edition, by Claire A.B. Freeland, PhD, and Jacqueline B. Toner, PhD; recommended for children aged 7 to 11 years
- *What to Do When You Worry Too Much: A Kid's Guide to Overcoming Anxiety*, 2nd Edition, by Dawn Huebner, PhD; recommended for children aged 6 to 12 years
- *What to Do When Your Brain Gets Stuck: A Kid's Guide to Overcoming OCD* by Dawn Huebner, PhD; recommended for children aged 6 to 12 years
- *When Harley Has Anxiety: A Fun CBT Skills Activity Book to Help Manage Worries and Fears* by Regine Galanti, PhD; recommended for children aged 5 to 9 years

Websites

- American Academy of Child and Adolescent Psychiatry—Anxiety and Children: www.aacap.org/AACAP/Families_and_Youth/Facts_for_Families/FFF-Guide/The-Anxious-Child-047.aspx
- American Psychological Association—Anxiety: www.apa.org/topics/anxiety
- Anxiety and Depression Association of America: https://adaa.org
- Child Mind Institute: https://childmind.org
- HealthyChildren.org—Mental Health Conditions: www.healthychildren.org/English/health-issues/conditions/emotional-problems/Pages/default.aspx
- National Institute of Mental Health: www.nimh.nih.gov
- Nemours TeensHealth: https://kidshealth.org/en/teens

••• Communication Pearl ••• Psychotherapy

- It is important to think of anxiety as a trait that runs in families.[11] Most often, parents, grandparents, and/or siblings may also struggle with anxiety. Helping families recognize a pattern may help reduce stigma around treatment.
- Anxiety often co-occurs with other behavioral health issues such as depression, attention-deficit/hyperactivity disorder (ADHD), autism spectrum disorder, and trauma/posttraumatic stress disorder.
- Parents may ask you for letters or notes for their children to get out of activities or tasks that cause them stress, such as sports, tests, and on-time arrival for school. Consider the potential impact of providing these types of accommodations, as they may contribute to the cycle of avoidance and cause more harm than good.[6] This can also apply to 504 plans for anxiety accommodations. For example, providing a letter that allows a child to show up to school late or take tests late (only for anxiety, not for other academic or behavioral concerns) may in fact exacerbate the problematic behavior.

Pharmacotherapy

In addition to psychotherapy, pharmacotherapy should be considered for patients with moderate anxiety, and it is recommended for patients with severe anxiety. Selective serotonin reuptake inhibitors (SSRIs) are considered first-line treatment, but serotonin-norepinephrine reuptake inhibitors (SNRIs) may also be used.[14,22] A helpful clinical pathway for the evaluation and treatment of patients at risk for anxiety can be found online (www.chop.edu/clinical-pathway/anxiety-and-ocd-clinical-pathway).

Other than for moderate or severe anxiety, other considerations for adding medication to the treatment plan include

- Interference with functioning that makes participation in psychotherapy challenging[14]
- Partial response to psychotherapy[14,22]
- Presence of comorbid mental health diagnoses[14]

➤ How should clinicians approach consent for medication management?

Engage the patient and family in a discussion about the risks and benefits of medication, as well as alternative options. Moving forward with medication management should happen as a mutual decision using the skills of shared decision-making with the patient and family. The informed consent of the patient differs depending on their developmental stage, but regardless of their ability to provide informed consent, the clinician will want to talk with the patient about starting a new medication and inquire about their understanding of medication management.

Discuss the US Food and Drug Administration (FDA) recommendations for close monitoring for suicidal ideation or behaviors during initiation and dose adjustments.[14] This includes also discussing the risks of not treating anxiety, which include suicidality.

➤ How should clinicians discuss SSRIs with patients?

- While there is evidence that SSRIs are safe and effective for pediatric anxiety, and are considered the first-line medication therapy, some of the SSRIs used are not FDA approved specifically for pediatric anxiety disorders.[23] However, they are used because there is ample evidence in the literature that these medications are safe and effective.[14,22,24,25] One SSRI, escitalopram, is FDA approved for children 7 years and older for the treatment of GAD.[23]
- Some SSRIs, such as sertraline and fluoxetine, are approved for other indications (ie, sertraline and fluoxetine for pediatric OCD; fluoxetine for pediatric depression) (refer to Chapter 11, Depression and Depressive Disorder, for more on depression treatment).[14,26] In addition to being used for anxiety, escitalopram is also FDA approved for the treatment of depression in adolescents.[23]

- Since sertraline and fluoxetine are FDA approved to treat OCD, they are also prescribed for anxiety disorders given some overlapping symptoms.[14,26]
- Frame what starting an SSRI might look like: daily medication, titration up, frequent monitoring, and tapering off when ready.
- Offer support: "The treatment team is here to help along the way and wants to communicate about any side effects, concerns, or symptoms." This includes sharing resources such as emergency lifelines (eg, 988).
- Ask if the patient and family have any questions and explain how they can follow up if they have new questions later.

Anxiety Pharmacotherapy

Fluoxetine and sertraline have the most evidence for the treatment of core anxiety disorders, although neither is FDA approved for anxiety disorders in children.[14,22,24,25] Escitalopram has FDA approval for children 7 years and older for the treatment of GAD.[23] Before starting any SSRI, it is important to look for drug-drug interactions with other medications a patient may be taking. Selective serotonin reuptake inhibitors may inhibit cytochrome P450 and should therefore be used with caution along with drugs that are metabolized by the CYP450 system.[27] Fluoxetine, sertraline, and escitalopram all come in tablet and solution forms. Overall, pediatric patients are more likely to experience adverse effects of SSRIs, so the general principle in initiating and titrating an SSRI is to "start low and go slow."[14,22,24] Table 10–1 gives general guidance on initiation, titration, and monitoring of SSRIs used for children and adolescents with anxiety.

Table 10–1. Suggested Dosing for Fluoxetine, Sertraline, and Escitalopram

Generic Name (Brand Name)	Initial Dosage	Titration	Max Daily Dose	Notes
Fluoxetine (Prozac)[a]	Children ≥7 years: 5–10 mg daily Adolescents: 10–20 mg daily	Children ≥7 years: 5 mg daily Adolescents: 10–20 mg daily	60 mg	• FDA approved for OCD in children ≥7 years and MDD in children ≥8 years • Typical dose range: children (5–10 mg), adolescents (10–40 mg) • Prolonged half-life, which helps prevent withdrawal symptoms if a dose is missed • Common adverse effects: nausea, headaches, weight reduction, abdominal pain

Continued on the next page

Table 10–1 (*continued*)

Generic Name (Brand Name)	Initial Dosage	Titration	Max Daily Dose	Notes
Sertraline (Zoloft)[b]	Children ≥6 years: 12.5–25 mg daily Adolescents: 25–50 mg daily	Children ≥6 years: 25 mg every 7 days, up to 100 mg Adolescents: 50 mg every 7 days, up to 100 mg	200 mg	• FDA approved for OCD in children ≥6 years • Typical dose range: children (25–100 mg), adolescents (50–150 mg) • Common adverse effects: gastrointestinal upset, headaches, insomnia
Escitalopram (Lexapro)[c]	Children ≥7 years: 5–10 mg daily	5–10 mg daily as clinically indicated after 2 weeks	20 mg	• FDA approved for GAD in children ≥7 years • Typical dose range: 10–20 mg • Common adverse effects: gastrointestinal upset, headaches, insomnia

Abbreviations: FDA, US Food and Drug Administration; GAD, generalized anxiety disorder; max, maximum; MDD, major depressive disorder; OCD, obsessive-compulsive disorder.

[a] Lexidrug. Fluoxetine: drug information. Retrieved March 18, 2026. https://online.lexi.com/lco/action/doc/retrieve/docid/chiphi_f/381212.

[b] Lexidrug. Sertraline: drug information. Retrieved March 18, 2026. https://online.lexi.com/lco/action/doc/retrieve/docid/chiphi_f/381448.

[c] Lexidrug. Escitalopram: drug information. Retrieved March 18, 2026. https://online.lexi.com/lco/action/doc/retrieve/docid/chiphi_f/4855723.

Adapted from Children's Hospital of Philadelphia. Medication management recommendations. Accessed February 18, 2026. https://www.chop.edu/clinical-pathway/anxiety-and-ocd-medication-management-recommendations#doses.

FDA-approved medication guides with more information on these medications can be found online (www.accessdata.fda.gov/scripts/cder/daf/index.cfm).

➤ What if a patient has multiple mental health diagnoses?

In general, treat the primary diagnosis, or the one with the most urgent or impairing symptoms, with an evidence-based medication.[14,22] For example, if a patient has anxiety and depression, fluoxetine is a good choice because it is FDA approved for depression and there is evidence in the literature for its effectiveness in treating anxiety.[14,22,24]

- Anxiety + depression → fluoxetine or escitalopram
- Anxiety + OCD → sertraline or fluvoxamine
- Anxiety + ADHD → sertraline

There is no clear evidence that one SSRI works better than another, but there are subtle differences.[14,22] Fluoxetine has a long half-life and can be more activating, which may be helpful for an adolescent with depressed and withdrawn behavior, but can sometimes be too activating for a younger child or a child with co-occurring ADHD or anxiety. Sertraline has a shorter half-life and can be divided into small doses. It also tends to be less activating, which can be helpful for younger, anxious patients.[14,26] At this time, there is no evidence that pharmacogenomic testing is effective in choosing an SSRI.[14]

When a first-line SSRI is not working or not tolerated, switching to an SNRI may be indicated. Box 10–3 gives an overview of an FDA approved SNRI for GAD.

Box 10-3. Serotonin-Norepinephrine Reuptake Inhibitors

These are considered second-line medications for anxiety management. Duloxetine (specifically Cymbalta) is most used because of its FDA approval for GAD.

Duloxetine (Cymbalta)[a]

- Children 7 years and older.
- Initial dose: 30 mg, may increase to 60 mg after 2 weeks.
- Typical dose: 30–60 mg.
- Titration: 30 mg every 2 weeks.
- Max dose: 120 mg daily.
- Common side effects: nausea, headache, weight reduction, abdominal pain.
- Rare potential serious side effects: serotonin syndrome, suicidal ideation, hepatic failure.
- Delayed-release capsules can be opened and sprinkled.

Abbreviations: FDA, US Food and Drug Administration; GAD, generalized anxiety disorder; max, maximum.

[a] Lexidrug. Duloxetine: drug information. Retrieved March 18, 2026. https://online.lexi.com/lco/action/doc/retrieve/docid/chiphi_f/6201017.

Adapted from Children's Hospital of Philadelphia. Medication management recommendations. Accessed February 18, 2026. https://www.chop.edu/clinical-pathway/anxiety-and-ocd-medication-management-recommendations#doses.

Counseling families about what to expect after starting an SSRI is important. While reviewing important monitoring parameters, including side effects, safety, and drug interactions, it is important to balance these concerns with optimism about the effectiveness of this treatment approach.

Keep in Mind: Adverse Effect Management

Many of the adverse effects of SSRIs go away after the first week or so of medication initiation or a dosage change.[14,24] If the symptoms are mild, remind patients that the symptoms should resolve and they should continue taking the medication. If the patient reports symptoms that are moderate to severe, consider discontinuing the medication with medical supervision.

- **Psychiatric adverse effects:** Activation of mania or hypomania. Because of this concern, it is important to screen for mania and hypomania before initiation and to ask about family history of bipolar disorder.[6,14] See Chapter 5, Somatic Symptoms and Depression, for tips on screening for psychosis and mania using questions such as "Do you ever have bursts of energy where you stay up all night doing things?" or "Do people ever tell you that you talk too much or too fast?"
- **Contraindications:** Patients taking a monoamine oxidate inhibitor (MAOI) should not take an SSRI. Caution and consideration should be used in patients with suspected bipolar disorder or mania, active substance use disorder, seizures, abnormal bleeding, hyponatremia, or glaucoma or those at risk for QT prolongation.[14,28]
- **Serotonin syndrome:** A toxicity of serotonin, which can be fatal, caused by too much serotonin in brain synapses resulting from drug interactions or overdose. Patients have a combination of neuromuscular, autonomic, and mental status symptoms. Symptoms concerning for serotonin syndrome include[29,30]
  - — Spontaneous clonus
  - — Agitation
  - — Diaphoresis
  - — Ocular clonus
  - — Tremor and hyperreflexia
  - — Hypertonia
  - — Fever with clonus

  Many drugs can precipitate serotonin toxicity by a variety of mechanisms. Patients at risk include those taking more than one SSRI/SNRI or taking high doses of these medications. Other potential precipitating drugs include meperidine, tramadol, pentazocine, metoclopramide, valproate, carbamazepine, dextromethorphan, cyclobenzaprine, trazodone, bupropion, and MAOIs (phenelzine, tranylcypromine, isocarboxazid, selegiline, linezolid, and methylene blue). Supplements such as St John's wort and tryptophan may also be implicated. Illegal drugs such as amphetamines, cocaine, MDMA (commonly referred to as "Ecstasy"), and levodopa are also risk factors.[29,30]

- **Black box warning:** All antidepressants, including the SSRIs, carry a black box warning that they could increase the risk for suicidal ideation for anyone 24 years or younger.[14,31] The black box warning exists because studies showed a small increase in incidence of suicidal thoughts, although not suicidal acts, with antidepressants compared to placebo.[10,31] Overall, the risk of an SSRI precipitating suicidal ideation is thought to be low, and there is a lot of evidence that SSRIs are safe to use in the pediatric population.[14,22,24,26,31] That said, it is important to assess for suicidal ideation before starting and while a patient is taking an SSRI, particularly around dosage changes, and to engage in basic safety planning with the patient and their family in case suicidal ideation develops.[14]
- **Safety planning:** A brief intervention in which the clinician and patient discuss individualized warning signs, coping strategies, and resources to use during a suicidal crisis.[14] This discussion can be documented through an online template (www.mysafetyplan.org) or an app (Stanley-Brown Safety Plan app) that the patient and caregiver have access to at home. (Refer to Chapter 9, Suicidality and Eating Disorder, and Chapter 11, Depression and Depressive Disorder, for more discussion on safety planning.)

••• Communication Pearl •••
How to Discuss the Black Box Warning With Parents and Caregivers

Clinicians can struggle with how to explain the black box warning to families, balancing the need for safety monitoring due to suicidal risk with a recommendation to use the medication to treat anxiety. Here is a sample script to explain the black box warning.

"Before we start an SSRI, I want to let you know that this medication has a black box warning from the FDA because it poses an increased risk for suicidal ideation while a young person is taking it. In studies, some young people taking SSRIs had a slight increase in suicidal thoughts but, importantly, not suicidal acts. Therefore, it is important that while your child is taking this medication, particularly in the beginning and with dosage changes, you monitor for any concerning changes in suicidal thoughts or behaviors. Please let me know if any suicidal thoughts develop. It's also important to have some other sources of help, like the Suicide & Crisis Lifeline (988), which you should keep in your phone as a quick reference. You can call or text this number 24/7 and someone trained will talk with you right away. It is important to remember, though, that although some children will have suicidal ideation while taking this medication, the risk is low. There are also risks for those with untreated anxiety. What questions do you have about this?"

- **Documentation:** The clinician should document the discussion that occurred between them and the patient/caregiver, including that they discussed the risks and benefits of treatment, including the black box warning. The plan should include the participation, understanding, and consent of the patient in a developmentally appropriate manner.

➤ Why are SSRIs titrated slowly?

Selective serotonin reuptake inhibitors may take 4 to 6 weeks to reach therapeutic effect.[14,22,24] An initial dose increase can be made after 2 to 4 weeks if the patient has been tolerating their starting dose. However, it is best to wait 4 to 8 weeks for subsequent dose increases to allow the medication to reach a steady state before assessing efficacy. It is important to explain to patients and caregivers that it takes 4 to 6 weeks to reach therapeutic effect of the medication, as this medication is different from many other medications they are familiar with (eg, pain relief, antibiotics) and patients may prematurely discontinue the medication, assuming it is not working.

Keep in Mind: "Start Low and Go Slow"

The starting dose is low so the clinician can observe for adverse effects. It takes 4 to 6 weeks for an SSRI to reach a steady state.[14,22,24] Begin the medication at the lowest effective dose to decrease the chance of adverse effects.

➤ What if a patient requests a medication to be taken as needed rather than daily?

While many patients and their families will request medications to be taken as needed for anxiety, in general this is not recommended. Medications in this category include diphenhydramine, hydroxyzine, and lorazepam. There is no evidence in the literature that these medications are effective for pediatric anxiety, and there is significant risk associated with them, including tolerance and dependence with benzodiazepines as well as sedation, dizziness, and incoordination with antihistamines.[11,12,14] Additionally, as-needed medication can be counterproductive to the goals of CBT. For example, if a patient takes an as-needed medication before an exposure, they are learning to take a medication instead of learning to gradually tolerate their anxiety.[11,12]

Follow-Up

During the medication initiation phase, follow-up appointments are typically scheduled, the first being within 1 to 2 weeks, to assess for adverse effects, including suicidal ideation.[14] Follow-ups typically continue weekly for the first 4 weeks. The follow-up evaluation can be done by a mental health specialist, the primary care clinician, or another team member. The follow-up schedule can be modified according to individual patient factors, and the patient's health record should include the clinical reasoning for the schedule chosen. It is appropriate to engage all care team members in the follow-up schedule and to make these appointments easily accessible to patients/families.

- Here is a general guideline for the medication initiation phase follow-up schedule.
  - First 4 weeks: weekly
  - Next 4 weeks: every 2 weeks
  - After 8 weeks: monthly or every few months as clinically indicated

Encourage family members to call immediately with any clinical concerns and to provide updates between appointments if needed. Families may also want to provide a HIPAA (Health Insurance Portability and Accountability Act) release so care team members can communicate with each other about the treatment plan and assess efficacy.

Treatment Resistance

In addition to reports from the patient and their family, use a rating scale to assess clinical response (if possible, the same scale used to make the initial diagnosis to compare scores over time). For anxiety, consider using the SCARED or GAD-7 (refer to Chapter 1, Somatic Symptoms or Panic Disorder).[14,32] The Children's Global Assessment Scale (CGAS) or Columbia Impairment Scale (CIS) can be used to assess a patient's functioning.[14] Refer to the Appendix for links to the tools online.

For patients with minimal or no response after 12 weeks of treatment, consider changing the treatment plan.[14,22] First, assess the patient's adherence to the medication and appropriate administration of each dose. If the patient confirms adherence and appropriate administration, next steps may include adding or changing psychotherapy or switching to another medication.

Titration Between Selective Serotonin Reuptake Inhibitors

- Switching from fluoxetine to sertraline: If the dose is higher than 40 mg, taper it; otherwise, stop fluoxetine, then wait 7 days for washout, and finally start sertraline at an initial dosage of 12.5 to 25 mg daily.
- Switching from sertraline to fluoxetine: Taper sertraline, then stop. Start a low dose (10 mg) of fluoxetine.

How quickly an SSRI is tapered depends on how high the dose is and how long a patient has been on it. In general, a slow taper is better and tapering the dose by 25% to 50% every month is a good overall guide. There is some evidence that a hyperbolic dose reduction rather than linear dose reduction is needed, especially at low doses near cessation to help mitigate withdrawal effects.[33] Some of the titration schedule is determined by what is feasible based on the medication formulation.

If the decision is made to switch the first SSRI to another SSRI, consider referring to an online tool (eg, https://switchrx.com) for titration guidance or consulting with a psychiatrist. For patients taking high doses or showing concerning side effects, urgent consultation with a psychiatrist or pediatric pharmacist may be necessary.

Discontinuing an SSRI

Discontinuation may be considered after a patient has achieved remission of anxiety symptoms for a period of 6 to 12 months and has not experienced functional impairment for at least 3 months.[14,22] Taper the medication over several months to reduce the risk for discontinuation syndrome (dizziness, fatigue, headaches, nausea, vomiting, insomnia, anxiety, and irritability).[14,24] During this phase and for several months after the patient is no longer taking the medication, monitor them for relapse of anxiety symptoms.[14,22]

Keep in Mind: Discontinuation Symptoms

Some adolescents will stop their SSRI on their own or wean more quickly than the clinician recommended. This self-management can result in discontinuation symptoms and have a flu-like presentation with symptoms including headache, diarrhea, nausea, vomiting, dizziness, or fatigue. When seeing patients with these symptoms who are taking an SSRI, the clinician should inquire about their medication adherence. Discontinuation symptoms are more common from medications with short half-lives, such as sertraline.[33]

When to Refer

The clinician should consider referring the patient to a pediatric psychiatrist in the following circumstances:

- Anytime they are uncomfortable with the management of the patient's anxiety or comorbidities
- Treatment resistance, or failure to improve after first-line medication
- Uncertain diagnosis
- Unusual medication side effects
- Polypharmacy complicating the treatment plan
- Multiple mental health comorbidities or a concern for mania or psychosis

Most states now have a telephonic psychiatric consultative service or child psychiatry access program that can be used by primary care clinicians for consultation, care coordination, and/or education and training programs (www.nncpap.org). Clinicians should become familiar with state-based resources. Examples of these resources include

- Massachusetts Child Psychiatry Access Project
- Commonwealth of Pennsylvania Telephonic Psychiatric Consultation Service Program
- California Child and Adolescent Mental Health Access Portal
- Virginia Mental Health Access Program

Discharge and Referral Back to the Primary Care Clinician

Patients' anxiety may be successfully comanaged by psychiatrists and primary care clinicians. Once the patient's condition seems stable, the psychiatrist may discharge the patient and the primary management of anxiety will return to the primary care clinician. Patients can be discharged when

- They are successfully weaned from the medication and there are no concerns for relapse.
- Their condition is stable with their medication and they need monitoring every 3 months for medication adherence, adverse effects, and anxiety symptom screening.
- If rating scales were used at baseline, repeated measures show significant decreases in total or subscale scores.

During the discharge process, discuss with the patient and their family the importance of ongoing monitoring of their mood and anxiety symptoms.[14,15] Anxiety symptoms can come in waves, and there may be a recurrence in the future, particularly around times involving stressors or life changes. Providing psychoeducation related to developmentally appropriate anxiety versus a relapse/recurrence is important, as well as reinforcing the skills and resources they already have in managing these symptoms. Patients and caregivers should understand when and where they should seek follow-up care for anxiety relapse/recurrence.

Lessons Learned About Anxiety and Anxiety Disorder Management and Initial Treatment

Anxiety is common in children and adolescents, and management involves a combination of psychotherapy and, if indicated, psychopharmacology.[15,24,26] Many patients will be able to receive comanaged or integrated care in primary care and with a therapist, but resistant or relapsing cases warrant further diagnostic exploration and often, comanagement with a psychiatrist.

- Medication is only one part of the treatment plan. Encourage lifestyle modifications, mindfulness/grounding/relaxation techniques, and psychotherapy.
- Cognitive behavioral therapy is evidence based for the treatment of anxiety.[11,12,14,15,24]
- Sertraline and fluoxetine are most often used to treat moderate to severe anxiety, but they do not have FDA approval for this indication.[11,15,24–26]
- Start low and go slow with initiation of an SSRI.
- Review the black box warning for SSRIs with patients and families.
- Avoid polypharmacy if possible.
- Make one change at a time and use rating scales to monitor symptoms and treatment response.

Keywords: anxiety, black box warning, CBT, GAD, OCD, serotonin syndrome, SNRI, SSRI

Suggested Reading

Oregon Psychiatric Access Line about Kids. *Mental Health Care Guide for Primary Care Clinicians: Anxiety.* Oregon Health & Science University; 2019. Accessed February 19, 2026. https://www.ohsu.edu/sites/default/files/2019-06/OPAL-K-Anxiety-Disorder-Care-Guide-2018.pdf

Riddle MA, Campo JV. Group 1 medications for anxiety and depression. In: *Pediatric Psychopharmacology for Primary Care.* 4th ed. American Academy of Pediatrics; 2025:105–124

References

1. Weitzman C, Guevara J, Curtin M, Macias M; American Academy of Pediatrics Section on Developmental and Behavioral Pediatrics, Council on Early Childhood, and Committee on Psychosocial Aspects of Child and Family Health; Society for Developmental and Behavioral Pediatrics. Promoting optimal development: screening for mental health, emotional, and behavioral problems: clinical report. *Pediatrics.* 2025;156(3):e2025073172 PMID: 40850690
2. Foy JM, Green CM, Earls MF; American Academy of Pediatrics Committee on Psychosocial Aspects of Child and Family Health, and Mental Health Leadership Work Group. Mental health competencies for pediatric practice. *Pediatrics.* 2019;144(5):e20192757 PMID: 31636143
3. Gray GV, Brody DS, Hart MT. Primary care and the de facto mental health care system: improving care where it counts. *Manag Care Interface.* 2000;13(3):62–65 PMID: 11066279
4. Cunningham PJ. Beyond parity: primary care physicians' perspectives on access to mental health care. *Health Aff (Millwood).* 2009;28(3):w490–w501 PMID: 19366722
5. Lee CM, Lutz J, Khau A, et al. Pediatric primary care perspectives of mental health services delivery during the COVID-19 pandemic. *Children (Basel).* 2022;9(8):1186 PMID: 36010056
6. American Psychiatric Association. Generalized anxiety disorder. In: *Diagnostic and Statistical Manual of Mental Disorders.* 5th ed, text rev. American Psychiatric Association Publishing; 2022:250–251
7. American Psychiatric Association. Social anxiety disorder (social phobia). In: *Diagnostic and Statistical Manual of Mental Disorders.* 5th ed, text rev. American Psychiatric Association Publishing; 2022:229–230
8. American Psychiatric Association. Separation anxiety disorder. In: *Diagnostic and Statistical Manual of Mental Disorders.* 5th ed, text rev. American Psychiatric Association Publishing; 2022:217
9. American Psychiatric Association. Panic disorder. In: *Diagnostic and Statistical Manual of Mental Disorders.* 5th ed, text rev. American Psychiatric Association Publishing; 2022:235–236
10. Compton SN, Walkup JT, Albano AM, et al. Child/Adolescent Anxiety Multimodal Study (CAMS): rationale, design, and methods. *Child Adolesc Psychiatry Ment Health.* 2010;4:1 PMID: 20051130
11. Kendall PC, Peterman JS. CBT for adolescents with anxiety: mature yet still developing. *Am J Psychiatry.* 2015;172(6):519–530 PMID: 26029805
12. Stiede JT, Trent ES, Viana AG, Guzick AG, Storch EA, Hershfield J. Cognitive behavioral therapy for children and adolescents with anxiety disorders. *Child Adolesc Psychiatr Clin N Am.* 2023;32(3):543–558 PMID: 37201966
13. Afshari B, Jafarian Dehkordi F, Asgharnejad Farid AA, et al. Study of the effects of cognitive behavioral therapy versus dialectical behavior therapy on executive function and reduction of symptoms in generalized anxiety disorder. *Trends Psychiatry Psychother.* 2022;44:e20200156 PMID: 35559733

14. Walter HJ, Bukstein OG, Abright AR, et al. Clinical practice guideline for the assessment and treatment of children and adolescents with anxiety disorders. *J Am Acad Child Adolesc Psychiatry.* 2020;59(10):1107–1124 PMID: 32439401
15. Wang Z, Whiteside SPH, Sim L, et al. Comparative effectiveness and safety of cognitive behavioral therapy and pharmacotherapy for childhood anxiety disorders: a systematic review and meta-analysis. *JAMA Pediatr.* 2017;171(11):1049–1056 PMID: 28859190
16. Davis TE III, May A, Whiting SE. Evidence-based treatment of anxiety and phobia in children and adolescents: current status and effects on the emotional response. *Clin Psychol Rev.* 2011;31(4):592–602 PMID: 21482318
17. Mohd Saat NZ, Hanawi SA, Hanafiah H, Ahmad M, Farah NMF, Abdul Rahman NAA. Relationship of screen time with anxiety, depression, and sleep quality among adolescents: a cross-sectional study. *Front Public Health.* 2024;12:1459952 PMID: 39678241
18. Munzer T, Parga-Belinkie J, Milkovich LM, et al; American Academy of Pediatrics Council on Communications and Media. Digital ecosystems, children, and adolescents. *Pediatrics.* 2026;157(2):e2025075320 PMID: 41556917
19. Riehm KE, Feder KA, Tormohlen KN, et al. Associations between time spend using social media and internalizing and externalizing problems among US youth. *JAMA Psychiatry.* 2019;76(12):1266–1273
20. Eirich R, McArthur BA, Anhorn C, McGuinness C, Christakis DA, Madigan S. Association of screen time with internalizing and externalizing behavior problems in children 12 years or younger: a systematic review and meta-analysis. *JAMA Psychiatry.* 2022;79(5):393–405 PMID: 35293954
21. Teague S, Somoray K, Shatte A, et al. Digital media use and child health and development: a systematic review and meta-analysis. *JAMA Pediatr.* 2026;e260085 PMID: 41801211
22. Walkup JT, Albano AM, Piacentini J, et al. Cognitive behavioral therapy, sertraline, or a combination in childhood anxiety. *N Engl J Med.* 2008;359(26):2753–2766 PMID: 18974308
23. Landy K, Rosani A, Esteves R. Escitalopram. In: *StatPearls.* StatPearls Publishing; 2026. Updated November 10, 2023. Accessed May 28, 2026. https://www.ncbi.nlm.nih.gov/books/NBK557734
24. Brawman-Mintzer O, Knapp RG, Rynn M, Carter RE, Rickels K. Sertraline treatment for generalized anxiety disorder: a randomized, double-blind, placebo-controlled study. *J Clin Psychiatry.* 2006;67(6):874–881 PMID: 16848646
25. Walkup JT, Labellarte MJ, Riddle MA, et al; Research Unit on Pediatric Psychopharmacology Anxiety Study Group. Fluvoxamine for the treatment of anxiety disorders in children and adolescents. *N Engl J Med.* 2001;344(17):1279–1285 PMID: 11323729
26. Pediatric OCD Treatment Study (POTS) Team. Cognitive-behavior therapy, sertraline, and their combination for children and adolescents with obsessive-compulsive disorder: the Pediatric OCD Treatment Study (POTS) randomized controlled trial. *JAMA.* 2004;292(16):1969–1976 PMID: 15507582
27. Hemeryck A, Belpaire FM. Selective serotonin reuptake inhibitors and cytochrome P-450 mediated drug-drug interactions: an update. *Curr Drug Metab.* 2002;3(1):13–37 PMID: 11876575
28. Lexidrug. Fluoxetine: drug information. Retrieved March 18, 2026. https://online.lexi.com/lco/action/doc/retrieve/docid/chiphi_f/381212
29. Foong AL, Grindrod KA, Patel T, Kellar J. Demystifying serotonin syndrome (or serotonin toxicity). *Can Fam Physician.* 2018;64(10):720–727 PMID: 30315014

30. Simon LV, Torrico TJ, Keenaghan M. Serotonin syndrome. In: *StatPearls*. StatPearls Publishing; 2025. Updated March 2, 2024. Accessed February 18, 2026. https://www.ncbi.nlm.nih.gov/books/NBK482377

31. US Food and Drug Administration. Class suicidality labeling language for antidepressants. 2005. Accessed May 28, 2026. https://www.accessdata.fda.gov/drugsatfda_docs/label/2005/21299s013lbl.pdf

32. Birmaher B, Brent DA, Chiappetta L, Bridge J, Monga S, Baugher M. Psychometric properties of the Screen for Child Anxiety Related Emotional Disorders (SCARED): a replication study. *J Am Acad Child Adolesc Psychiatry*. 1999;38(10):1230–1236 PMID: 10517055

33. Sørensen A, Juhl Jørgensen K, Munkholm K. Clinical practice guideline recommendations on tapering and discontinuing antidepressants for depression: a systematic review. *Ther Adv Psychopharmacol*. 2022;12:20451253211067656 PMID: 35173954

CHAPTER 11

Depression and Depressive Disorder

Treatment of patients with subthreshold depressive symptoms or depressive disorders can be initiated in the pediatric primary care setting. The American Academy of Pediatrics (AAP) endorses that to promote the optimal development of children, behavioral and emotional screening should happen routinely in pediatric primary care so early intervention can occur.[1] Pediatric clinicians are well positioned to address the behavioral and mental health of their patients because of their longitudinal relationships with patients and their families, whole-child approach, and ability to initiate treatment and/or serve as a bridge to mental health specialists.[2]

Screening for depression, diagnosis of depression, and assessment of depression severity were discussed in the cases in Chapters 5, Somatic Symptoms and Depression; 6, Depression of Chronic Disease; and 9, Suicidality and Eating Disorder. Some cases presented subthreshold depressive symptoms that caused impairment in functioning but did not rise to the level of a clinical diagnosis, while others met criteria for a disorder and required a higher level of clinical and medical intervention. It is important to understand the difference between the two to find the best avenue for care and management in the clinical setting. Feeling sad and changes in mood will ebb and flow, especially during adolescence, and should not always be pathologized but rather used as context clues to understand how these symptoms interfere with a person's functioning. Thus, helping patients distinguish between managing symptoms and managing a disorder is an important distinction. While diagnostic criteria for depressive disorders will be reviewed, the purpose of this chapter is to review psychoeducation, psychotherapy, medication management, referral to psychologists and/or psychiatrists, and the comanagement of patients with depression.

When discussing treatment options for depression with a patient, it is important to provide the patient with psychoeducation about depression, including its impact on functioning; evidence-based treatment options; medication options (if applicable); and brief interventions to help maintain and stabilize the patient's mood and functioning in one's role as the primary care clinician.

Keep in Mind: A Primary Care Clinician's Role

- Facilitate brief interventions in the office, including evidence-based screening tools.
- Initiate first-line medications as clinically indicated.
- Provide referrals to mental health specialists.
- Provide supportive monitoring until a mental health specialist is involved and the patient's condition is stable with medication

Review the Diagnostic Criteria for Depressive Disorders

In a perfect world, a clinician would be able to use a brief screening tool and then refer a patient for follow-up intervention if a diagnostic evaluation were warranted. However, because of pediatric mental health specialist shortages or extended wait times for appointments, pediatric primary care clinicians often need to manage their patient's mental health care issues.[3–5] Therefore, it is important for these clinicians to understand how to assess for conditions like depressive disorders. As always, seek consultation and team-based collaboration with mental health specialists whenever possible.

To assess for depression issues and potential depressive disorders, use a clinical interview (eg, with patient and multiple raters such as parents/caregivers and schools/teachers); criteria from the *Diagnostic and Statistical Manual of Mental Disorders, Fifth Edition, Text Revision* (*DSM-5-TR*); and brief, standardized screening tools (eg, Patient Health Questionnaire-9 Modified for Adolescents [PHQ-A]), in addition to assessment of functional impairment to make a diagnosis of depression.[6] Refer to the Appendix for a description and link to the tool online. A typical depression diagnosis in pediatric primary care includes

Major depressive disorder (MDD)[7]: Diagnosed when a person has 5 or more symptoms nearly every day over a 2-week period. These symptoms should be a change from baseline.

- At least 1 of the following symptoms must be present:
  - — Low or depressed mood
  - — Diminished interest or pleasure in activities
- Other symptoms can include
  - — Weight loss or decreased appetite
  - — Insomnia or hypersomnia
  - — Psychomotor agitation or retardation
  - — Fatigue or loss of energy
  - — Feelings of worthlessness or guilt
  - — Difficulty concentrating
  - — Either recurrent thoughts of death or suicidal ideation/attempt

This chapter focuses on MDD, which is the most common diagnosis in children and adolescents.

Keep in Mind: Depression Is Not One Diagnosis

Major depressive disorder is just one of the depressive disorders classified in the *DSM-5-TR*. Other diagnoses include persistent depressive disorder, disruptive mood dysregulation disorder, premenstrual dysphoric disorder, substance/medication-induced depressive disorder, depressive disorder caused by another medical condition, and other specified/unspecified depressive disorders.[7] While this chapter discusses MDD, it is important to understand the difference between the classifications. Additionally, you are likely to encounter subthreshold depression, particularly with preteens and adolescents. The word "depressed" is common vernacular for feeling sad and moody and does not necessarily indicate a disorder unless specific criteria is met.

Psychoeducation

Everyone has low mood or depressive symptoms on occasion, but these can be tricky to discuss with youth and families, because the word "depression" is common vernacular used to describe labile and transient moods typically synonymous with the ups and downs of life. However, proper identification, early detection, and support are crucial aspects to minimize the impact that depressive symptoms can have on overall functioning. Some key talking points to use when discussing depressive symptoms with patients include

- Keep language simple and clear, especially when talking with younger children. Consider using metaphors or describing symptoms in more child-friendly language. For example,
  — "Sometimes our brain gets tired, just like our body. When our brain gets tired, we may feel sad."
  — "Sometimes we may not want to do things we normally love to do, like hanging out with friends or playing at the park, because they feel like too much effort. Have you felt like that?"
  — "Depression can sometimes feel like a heavy backpack, filled with books, that is glued to your body, and you can't take it off. Have you ever felt like that?"
- Build a therapeutic alliance with the patient and family by displaying empathy, normalizing feelings, and empowering patients to speak about their feelings. The HEL^{2}P^3 mnemonic, developed by the AAP Task Force on Mental Health, can be used to build trust and develop a plan of care.[2]
  — H = Hope.
  — E = Empathy.
  — L^2 = Language, Loyalty.
  — P^3 = Permission, Partnership, Plan.

- Try to use open-ended questions that go beyond yes/no answers, such as "What are some sad thoughts you have?" instead of "Do you have sad thoughts?"
- Validate feelings as much as possible: "I feel honored that you shared that with me. It must have felt hard to say that out loud, and I'm here to help you feel better."
- Acknowledge to caregivers that it can be difficult to hear their child talk about depressive symptoms and that it is OK to feel overwhelmed, but now everyone is on the same team to help their child feel better.
- Make sure to emphasize strengths in the child and family whenever possible.

Depression management varies based on severity and may include psychotherapy alone, psychotherapy and pharmacotherapy, and, sometimes also, a referral to a higher level of care, as explained in **Box 11-1**.[6,8,9]

Box 11-1. Depression Management by Severity[a]

- **Mild:** psychotherapy alone
- **Moderate:** psychotherapy + pharmacotherapy
- **Severe:** psychotherapy + pharmacotherapy + consideration of referral for a higher level of care

[a] March J, Silva S, Petrycki S, et al; Treatment for Adolescents With Depression Study (TADS) Team. Fluoxetine, cognitive-behavioral therapy, and their combination for adolescents with depression: Treatment for Adolescents With Depression Study (TADS) randomized controlled trial. *JAMA*. 2004;292(7):807–820.

Evidence-Based Treatment Options

The Treatment for Adolescents With Depression Study (TADS)[9] was a multisite randomized controlled trial that evaluated the effectiveness of fluoxetine alone, cognitive behavioral therapy (CBT) alone, and their combination in adolescents with MDD. In this study, the administration of fluoxetine was double blinded for the first 12 weeks. The TADS showed that

- Fluoxetine combined with CBT was most effective early on. Fluoxetine alone or combined with CBT accelerates improvement relative to CBT alone (**Box 11-2**).
- Adding CBT to fluoxetine minimizes suicidal ideation and events.

Therefore, in response to the TADS, adolescents with moderate to severe depression are often treated initially with a combination of fluoxetine and CBT rather than either alone.[9,10]

Abbreviations: CBT, cognitive behavioral therapy; SSRI, selective serotonin reuptake inhibitor.

Box 11-2. Treatment for Adolescents With Depression Study[a,b]

- Twelve weeks: CBT + SSRI > SSRI > CBT.
- 36 weeks: CBT = SSRI = CBT + SSRI.
- One year: Treatment benefits continued.

At 12 weeks, combination treatment with CBT and fluoxetine (SSRI) showed the best response, but by 36 weeks, all groups showed similar improvement. The benefits of treatment continued 1 year after treatment ended.

[a] March J, Silva S, Petrycki S, et al; Treatment for Adolescents With Depression Study (TADS) Team. Fluoxetine, cognitive-behavioral therapy, and their combination for adolescents with depression: Treatment for Adolescents With Depression Study (TADS) randomized controlled trial. *JAMA*. 2004;292(7):807–820.

[b] March JS, Vitiello B. Clinical messages from the Treatment for Adolescents With Depression Study (TADS). *Am J Psychiatry*. 2009;166(10):1118–1123.

Psychotherapy

There are specific evidence-based psychotherapy recommendations for depression.[11–13] Refer to these therapies by name when discussing them with the patient and family.

- **Cognitive behavioral therapy (CBT):** focuses on identifying and challenging negative thought patterns and their resulting behaviors
  - There is another type of CBT known as trauma-focused cognitive behavioral therapy (TF-CBT), which uses the same components of CBT with a trauma-focused lens to reduce the symptoms of trauma and posttraumatic stress. It can be helpful for co-occurring depression, anxiety, and other behavioral issues stemming from trauma.[14]
- **Interpersonal psychotherapy for adolescents (IPT-A):** focuses on improving interpersonal relationships and conflicts that contribute to and can manifest depressive symptoms
- **Dialectical behavior therapy for adolescents (DBT-A):** focuses on emotion regulation, distress tolerance, mindfulness, and interpersonal effectiveness
- **Acceptance and commitment therapy (ACT):** focuses on the acceptance of emotions and behaviors and uses tools such as mindfulness to help change negative thoughts

Family-focused therapy approaches and group therapy can also be helpful modalities depending on context. Group therapy may be preferred by teens, as it can help them feel socially connected and less alone.

••• Communication Pearl •••
Psychotherapy

There are many ways a patient might seek therapy, and there are many types of therapists—from master's-level clinicians (eg, marriage and family therapists, licensed professional counselors), to licensed clinical social workers, to doctoral-level psychologists (eg, PhD, PsyD). It's important to help caregivers understand how big the therapeutic world can be as they strive to choose a practitioner for their child or family. All therapists have different theoretical orientations that guide their practice and may not align with evidence-based treatment or gold standards. Additionally, there may be difficulties in obtaining specific types of therapies because of barriers related to availability/waiting lists, insurance/out-of-pocket costs, transportation, etc. While we will always recommend evidence-based therapies to address a behavioral health concern, there is research-based evidence to suggest that most psychotherapy treatments can produce beneficial outcomes and that the quality of the relationship is important.[15,16]

Therefore, it is vital for a child/teen to feel connected to their therapist, even if not specifically trained in CBT/IPT-A/DBT-A/ACT. However, choosing a therapist trained in one of these modalities should ensure progress, as these interventions are founded on research that demonstrates favorable outcomes for symptom improvement.

Last, remind patients and families that their first therapist might not be the right fit, but that does not mean that therapy does not work or that they should give up finding the right therapist for them. A metaphor we sometimes use with families is to think of therapist fit like a pair of jeans: not all jeans are the same, even from the same company and the same size. There are different types of fabrics, styles, lengths, etc, so it is necessary to try them on to see how they fit but not get discouraged if you need to keep looking for the right one.

Brief Interventions and Continuity of Care

It is important to maintain a connection with patients and their families while they seek treatment or wait for an appointment. The clinician can suggest quick, active, and simple strategies that can help address the cognitive and somatic impairments of depression. Consider using strategies that involve healthy habits or lifestyle modifications; behavioral activation; emotion regulation skills and problem-solving; and cognitive restructuring.

Healthy Habits/Lifestyle Modifications

- Focus on improving sleep hygiene, as research suggests that sleep disturbances (eg, more wakefulness in bed, lighter sleep, prolonged sleep, and multiple wakings) can act as a precursor to the development of depression.[17]
- Limit screen time to help increase physical activity, promote social/family interaction, and inhibit impact on sleep hygiene.[18,19]

- Increase physical activity and social interactions.
- Eat healthy meals and ensure that caloric intake goals are met daily.
- Limit/monitor social media use. Research has shown that greater social media use is significantly associated with internalizing problems, including anxiety and depression.[20–22]

Behavioral Activation

- Behavioral activation is often a first step in the treatment of depression. Encourage the patient to identify a fun activity, then create a plan or work with the patient to problem-solve for them to complete that task (refer to the Emotion Regulation Skills and Problem-Solving section later in this chapter). By engaging in simple, pleasant activities, it is possible to improve mood and energy levels. Ideal activities are those that are social and will allow the individual to feel accomplished after completing the activity (eg, reading a chapter in a book, cleaning, or organizing).
- Encourage patients to make a list of pleasant activities and ask them to commit to trying 1 or 2 before their next check-in appointment. Examples include
  - Writing in a journal
  - Watching a sunset/sunrise
  - Going rock climbing
  - Visiting neighbors/friends
  - Volunteering
  - Playing a sport

Emotion Regulation Skills and Problem-Solving

- Emotion regulation: Mindfulness can help youth learn to pay attention to the present moment, including thoughts, feelings, and body sensations. The clinician should listen with openness and without judgment. Explain how mindfulness can help youth realize negative thoughts without letting them ruminate and affect their mood and behavior.[23]
- Problem-solving skills
  - Introduce a step-by-step method to problem-solving, as youth with depressive symptoms typically struggle to initiate tasks because of their mood.[24] Tackling 1 step at a time can help individuals feel less stuck and more in control of the situation.
    - Step 1: Define the problem.
    - Step 2: Brainstorm solutions.
    - Step 3: Evaluate options.
    - Step 4: Try 1 of the options and review.

Cognitive Restructuring

- Depressive symptoms can produce unhelpful thinking styles. The way people think can affect the way they feel and behave. Discuss the importance of challenging negative thoughts. Refer to the following sample conversation for examples of how to challenge a patient's negative thoughts about feeling excluded from their friend group:

Clinician: What is the negative thought you are having?

Patient: All my friends hate me and I'm a loser.

Clinician: Is there any evidence to the thought? Is there opposing evidence?

Patient: I actually have a good group of friends, but no one is answering my calls or liking my photos on Instagram.

Clinician: What would a friend think about this situation?

Patient: It's a little weird and I can see why you think that, but I'm just busy and I didn't see it. I had 2 softball games this weekend.

Clinician: Is there a different way to look at the situation or think about it now?

Patient: My friends are just busy, or they didn't see my post.

Clinician: What would be a helpful thought to have about this same situation in the future?

Patient: My friends just must be busy. I'll listen to some music and call them again. It's OK.

For patients who are being referred to a mental health specialist, the strategies described in this section can be initiated to offer them some tools to address depressive thoughts while they await therapy. These strategies are equally useful for symptoms that present during stressful patient care encounters. Educate patients and families about other resources, such as apps, books/workbooks, or websites, that they can use to build skills and feel more confident in managing depressive symptoms at home. Many of these resources use some of the same approaches and techniques that patients will learn in psychotherapy and can be a helpful bridge for improving daily functioning until they establish care with their mental health specialist.

Resources

Crisis and Support/Suicide Lines

- 988 Suicide & Crisis Lifeline: Call or text 988 or start a chat through https://chat.988lifeline.org.
- Crisis Text Line: Text HELLO or HOLA to 741741 or start a chat through https://connect.crisistextline.org/chat.
- Call 911 or visit the nearest emergency department.

Apps

We expect technology to change over time and encourage readers to find apps endorsed by groups such as the American Academy of Pediatrics, the American Psychological Association, and the American Academy of Child and Adolescent Psychiatry. Clinicians can work with families to identify apps that may be helpful for their specific needs.

Books

- *Conquer Negative Thinking for Teens: A Workbook to Break the Nine Thought Habits That Are Holding You Back* by Mary Karapetian Alvord, PhD, and Anne McGrath, MA
- *Freeing Your Child From Negative Thinking: Powerful, Practical Strategies to Build a Lifetime of Resilience, Flexibility, and Happiness* by Tamar Chansky, PhD
- *How to Get Unstuck From the Negative Muck: A Kid's Guide to Getting Rid of Negative Thinking* by Lake Sullivan, PhD
- *Rescuing Your Teenager from Depression* by Norman T. Berlinger, MD, PhD
- *The Teenage Brain: Understanding Anxiety and Depression in Teenagers; A Guide for Parents, Counselors and Teens* by Kasey P. Crist, LMHC

Websites

- American Academy of Child and Adolescent Psychiatry—Depression in Children and Teens: www.aacap.org/AACAP/Families_and_Youth/Facts_for_Families/FFF-Guide/The-Depressed-Child-004.aspx
- American Psychological Association—Depression Treatments for Children and Adolescents: www.apa.org/depression-guideline/children-and-adolescents
- Anxiety and Depression Association of America: https://adaa.org
- Child Mind Institute: https://childmind.org
- HealthyChildren.org—Mental Health Conditions: www.healthychildren.org/English/health-issues/conditions/emotional-problems/Pages/default.aspx
- National Institute of Mental Health: www.nimh.nih.gov
- Nemours TeensHealth: https://kidshealth.org/en/teens
- Seize the Awkward: https://seizetheawkward.org

Pharmacotherapy

Pharmacotherapy should be considered for patients with moderate to severe depression.[9,10,25] Using pharmacotherapy in addition to psychotherapy, specifically CBT, improves treatment response and safety.[9,10,25] Selective serotonin reuptake inhibitors (SSRIs) are first-line treatment, but serotonin-norepinephrine reuptake inhibitors (SNRIs) may also be used.[25] Both fluoxetine and escitalopram are US Food and Drug Administration (FDA)–approved treatments for children and adolescents with depression, starting at age 8 years for fluoxetine and age 12 years for escitalopram.[26,27] A helpful clinical pathway for the evaluation and treatment of patients at risk for depression can be found online (www.chop.edu/clinical-pathway/depression-clinical-pathway).

➤ How should clinicians approach consent for medication management?

Engage the patient and family in a discussion about the risks and benefits of medication, as well as alternative options. Moving forward with medication management should happen as a mutual decision using the skills of shared decision-making with the patient and family. The informed consent of the patient differs depending on their developmental stage, but regardless of their ability to provide informed consent, the clinician will want to talk with the patient about starting a new medication and inquire about their understanding of medication management.

Discuss the FDA recommendations for close monitoring for suicidal ideation or behaviors during initiation and dose adjustments.[25,28] This includes also discussing the risks of not treating depression, which include suicidality.[7,25]

➤ How should clinicians discuss SSRIs with patients?

- Ask patients what they know about depression, then explain how depression is a medical illness just like other illnesses they know about, such as asthma or eczema.
- Focus on how depression is causing negative symptoms for them and that the medication may help improve these.
- Explain that moderate to severe depression does not go away on its own and patients need treatment to get better or symptoms can worsen over time.[9]
- Discuss what SSRIs are and how they increase the level of the chemical messenger serotonin in the brain.
- Frame what starting an SSRI might look like: daily medication, titration up, frequent monitoring, and tapering off when ready.
- Offer support: "The treatment team is here to help along the way and wants to communicate about any side effects, concerns, or symptoms." This includes sharing resources such as emergency lifelines (eg, 988).
- Ask if they have any questions, and explain how they can follow up if they have new questions later.

Keep in Mind: "Start Low and Go Slow"

The starting dose is low so the clinician can observe for adverse effects. It takes 4 to 6 weeks for an SSRI to reach a steady state. Begin the medication at the lowest effective dose to decrease the chance of adverse effects.

Depression Pharmacotherapy

Fluoxetine and escitalopram are FDA approved for depression and have the most evidence in children and adolescents.[26–29] Both fluoxetine and escitalopram come in tablet and oral solution forms. Some SSRIs may inhibit cytochrome P450 and should therefore be used with caution along with drugs that are metabolized by the CYP450 system.[30] **Table 11-1** gives general guidance on initiation, titration, and monitoring of SSRIs used for children and adolescents with depression.

Table 11-1. Suggested Dosing for Fluoxetine and Escitalopram

Generic Name (Brand Name)	Initial Dosage	Titration	Max Daily Dose	Notes
Fluoxetine (Prozac)[a]	Children ≥7 years: 5–10 mg daily Adolescents: 10–20 mg daily	Children ≥7 years: 5 mg daily Adolescents: 10–20 mg daily	60 mg	• FDA approved for OCD in children ≥7 years and MDD in children ≥ 8 years • Typical dose range: children (5–10 mg), adolescents (10–40 mg) • Prolonged half-life, which helps prevent withdrawal symptoms if a dose is missed • Common adverse effects: nausea, headaches, weight reduction, abdominal pain
Escitalopram (Lexapro)[b]	Children ≥7 years: 5–10 mg daily	5–10 mg daily as clinically indicated after 2 weeks	20 mg	• FDA approved for GAD in children ≥7 years • Typical dose range: 10–20 mg • Common adverse effects: gastrointestinal upset, headaches, insomnia

Abbreviations: FDA, US Food and Drug Administration; GAD, generalized anxiety disorder; max, maximum; MDD, major depressive disorder; OCD, obsessive-compulsive disorder.

[a] Lexidrug. Fluoxetine: drug information. Retrieved March 18, 2026. https://online.lexi.com/lco/action/doc/retrieve/docid/chiphi_f/381212.

[b] Lexidrug. Escitalopram: drug information. Retrieved March 18, 2026. https://online.lexi.com/lco/action/doc/retrieve/docid/chiphi_f/4855723.

Adapted from Children's Hospital of Philadelphia. Medication management recommendations. Accessed February 18, 2026. https://www.chop.edu/clinical-pathway/anxiety-and-ocd-medication-management-recommendations#doses.

FDA-approved medication guides with more information on these medications can be found online (www.accessdata.fda.gov/scripts/cder/daf/index.cfm).

- **Psychiatric adverse effects:** Activation of mania or hypomania. Because of this concern, it is important to screen for mania and hypomania before initiation and to ask about family history of bipolar disorder. See Chapter 5, Somatic Symptoms and Depression, for tips on screening for psychosis and mania using questions such as "Do you ever have bursts of energy where you stay up all night doing things?" or "Do people ever tell you that you talk too much or too fast?"
- **Contraindications:** Patients taking a monoamine oxidate inhibitor (MAOI) should not take an SSRI.[29] Caution and consideration should be used in patients with suspected bipolar disorder or mania, active substance use disorder, seizures, abnormal bleeding, hyponatremia, or glaucoma or in those at risk for QT prolongation.[6,28]
- **Serotonin syndrome:** A toxicity of serotonin, which can be fatal, caused by too much serotonin in brain synapses resulting from drug interactions or overdose. Patients have a combination of neuromuscular, autonomic, and mental status symptoms. Symptoms concerning for serotonin syndrome include[31,32]
  - Spontaneous clonus
  - Agitation
  - Diaphoresis
  - Ocular clonus
  - Tremor and hyperreflexia
  - Hypertonia
  - Fever with clonus

  Many drugs can precipitate serotonin toxicity by a variety of mechanisms. Patients at risk include those taking more than one SSRI/SNRI or taking high doses of these medications. Other potential precipitating drugs include meperidine, tramadol, pentazocine, metoclopramide, valproate, carbamazepine, dextromethorphan, cyclobenzaprine, trazodone, bupropion, and MAOIs (phenelzine, tranylcypromine, isocarboxazid, selegiline, linezolid, and methylene blue). Supplements such as St John's wort and tryptophan may also be implicated. Illegal drugs such as amphetamines, cocaine, MDMA (commonly referred to as "Ecstasy"), and levodopa are also risk factors.[28,33]
- **Black box warning:** All antidepressants, including the SSRIs, carry a black box warning that they could increase the risk for suicidal ideation for anyone 24 years or younger.[7,9,10] The black box warning exists because studies showed a small increase in incidence of suicidal thoughts, although not suicidal acts, with antidepressants compared to placebo.[10,28] Overall, the risk of an SSRI precipitating suicidal ideation is thought to be low, and there is a lot of evidence that SSRIs are safe to use in the pediatric population.[25–27] That said, it is important to assess for suicidal ideation before starting and while a patient is taking an SSRI, particularly around dose changes, and to engage in safety planning with a patient and their family in case suicidal ideation develops.[34]

••• Communication Pearl •••
How to Discuss the Black Box Warning With Parents and Caregivers

Clinicians can struggle with how to explain the black box warning to families, balancing the need for safety monitoring due to suicidal risk with a recommendation to use the medication to treat depression. Here is a sample script to explain the black box warning.

"Before we start an SSRI, I want to let you know that this medication has a black box warning from the FDA because it poses an increased risk for suicidal ideation while a young person is taking it. In studies, some young people taking SSRIs had a slight increase in suicidal thoughts but, importantly, not suicidal acts. Therefore, it is important that while your child is taking this medication, particularly in the beginning and with dosage changes, you monitor for any concerning changes in suicidal thoughts or behaviors. Please let me know if any suicidal thoughts develop. It's also important to have some other sources of help, like the Suicide & Crisis Lifeline (988), which you should keep in your phone as a quick reference. You can call or text this number 24/7 and someone trained will talk with you right away. It is important to remember, though, that although some children will have suicidal ideation while taking this medication, the risk is low. There are also risks for those with untreated depression. What questions do you have about this?"

- **Safety planning:** All patients diagnosed with depression should have a safety plan in place. Nearly half of all people who die by suicide have a known mental health diagnosis, with depression being the most common.[34] Depression screening tools often contain questions related to suicide, so providing these frequently during routine visits and follow-ups can help identify potential suicidal ideation. Best practices now suggest screening for suicide and safety planning as a component of every medical visit.[1,6] The more frequently the clinician poses these questions, the greater the likelihood of normalizing these emotions and identifying them promptly. Once suicidal ideation is identified, it is important to create and implement a safety plan.[8] Key steps in creating a safety plan include
  - — Assess immediate risk: Is this patient in imminent danger of hurting or killing themselves or others? Is there a current plan or intent? Are they safe to return home?
  - — Have a calm conversation about the importance of creating a safety plan, using clear, nonjudgmental, nonclinical language.
  - — Collaboratively create the plan using the Stanley-Brown Safety Plan (Refer to Chapter 9, Suicidality and Eating Disorder, for more information on safety planning.)
  - — Involve parents/caregivers with patient consent unless doing so will cause harm. Be sure to discuss how to make the environment safe, including restricting access to lethal items (eg, locking away knives and medication, removing razor blades or other sharp objects).

- Document the plan (both in writing and in the electronic health record) and provide a copy to the patient.
- Create a plan to follow up and/or help the family connect with an appropriate level of care.

- **Documentation:** The clinician should document the discussion that occurred between them and the patient/caregiver, including that they discussed the risks and benefits of treatment, including the black box warning. The plan should include the participation, understanding, and consent of the patient in a developmentally appropriate manner.

➤ How many patients get better with treatment?

Approximately 60% of adolescents will respond to initial treatment with either an antidepressant medication or an evidence-based method of psychotherapy (CBT or IPT-A).[9,10] An adequate clinical response is defined as a 50% reduction in symptoms.[6,9] An adequate trial of medication is 8 weeks with at least 4 weeks at a therapeutic dose.[10] When a patient does not seem to respond to treatment,

- Ensure adherence to the medication.
- Inquire about psychotherapy: Is it CBT or IPT-A? How often do they attend therapy?
- Maximize the dose to the therapeutic window before making a change in medication.[2,9,10]

➤ What if a patient has multiple mental health diagnoses?

In general, treat the primary diagnosis, or the one with the most urgent or impairing symptoms, with an evidence-based medication.[6] For example, if a patient has anxiety and depression, fluoxetine or escitalopram is a good choice, depending on age, because both are FDA approved for depression, escitalopram is approved for GAD, and there is evidence in the literature for their effectiveness in treating anxiety.[9,26]

There is no clear evidence that one SSRI works better than another, but there are subtle differences.[27,33] Fluoxetine has a long half-life and can be more activating, which may be helpful for an adolescent with a depressed and withdrawn mood, but can sometimes be too activating for a younger child or a child with coexisting ADHD or anxiety. Sertraline has a shorter half-life and can be divided into small doses. It also tends to be less activating, which can be helpful for younger patients with low mood.[28]

➤ What is treatment-resistant depression?

Treatment-resistant depression or depression recurrence is more common when there is/are[10,35,36]

- Earlier age of onset
- Increased severity of episodes

- Psychosocial stressors
- Genetic history
- Family conflict
- Coexisting conditions, such as anxiety, substance use disorder, or eating disorders

Patients with treatment-resistant depression experience an increased risk for suicidality, so close monitoring and screening are recommended.[25,36] Refer to Chapter 9, Suicidality and Eating Disorder, for more information on suicidality.

If depression is chronic, further medical workup may be indicated. Components to consider include

- Performing laboratory evaluation[37]
  - Complete blood cell count
  - Thyrotropin (previously referred to as *thyroid-stimulating hormone*) level
  - Vitamin B_{12} and folate levels
  - Urine toxicology
  - Vitamin D level
  - C-reactive protein level
- Exploring the differential diagnosis for chronic illnesses associated with increased rates of depression[37]
  - Neurological diseases
    - Epilepsy
    - Migraines
    - Complex regional pain syndrome
  - Allergic diseases
    - Asthma
    - Eczema
    - Food allergies
  - Inflammatory disorders
    - Systemic lupus erythematosus
    - Inflammatory bowel disease
    - Celiac disease
    - Psoriasis
  - School-related concerns
    - Learning disability
    - Bullying
  - Trauma history
    - Past traumatic events or adverse childhood events
  - Endocrine disorders
    - Hashimoto disease (chronic lymphocytic thyroiditis)
    - Diabetes

- Asking about medications that might increase the risk for depression or cause symptoms of depression[37]
  - β-Blockers
  - Antihistamines
  - Steroids
  - Antiepileptic drugs
  - Interferon
  - Oral contraceptives

While switching to another SSRI or adding psychosocial interventions is recommended for treatment-resistant depression, consider referring to or consulting with a psychiatrist in these cases. If a patient does not respond to 2 SSRIs, alternative antidepressant therapies may be used but are not approved by the FDA for the treatment of depression in youth and should be done in consultation with a psychiatrist.

Follow-Up

During the medication initiation phase, follow-up appointments are typically scheduled, the first being within 1 to 2 weeks, to assess for adverse effects, including suicidal ideation.[28] Follow-ups typically continue weekly for the first 4 weeks. The follow-up evaluation can be done by a mental health specialist, the primary care clinician, or another team member. The follow-up schedule can be modified according to individual patient factors, and the patient's health record should include the clinical reasoning for the schedule chosen. It is appropriate to engage all care team members in the follow-up schedule and to make these appointments easily accessible to patients/families.

- Here is a general guideline for the medication initiation phase follow-up schedule.
  - First 4 weeks: weekly
  - Next 4 weeks: every 2 weeks
  - After 8 weeks: monthly or every few months as clinically indicated

The clinician may want to see the patient off cycle to assess their symptom severity during times when there are known stressors or challenges. In many cases, these include times of transition (eg, back to school, graduation, college entry), family stressors (eg, marriages, divorces, new birth), or social stressors (eg, SATs, prom, college application deadlines). It is a good idea to make caregivers aware of how some of these stressors or challenges may trigger a flare of symptoms, so they can be vigilant at these times and monitor at home for symptoms or behavioral changes.

➤ How often should the patient be rescreened?

Rescreen the patient every 2 to 3 months with the same tools that were originally used to make the diagnosis to assess treatment success and monitor for remission.

Discontinuing an SSRI

Selective serotonin reuptake inhibitors have a hyperbolic dose-response relationship, which means that at smaller doses, the changes to the serotonin receptor are greater; therefore, there are more severe withdrawal symptoms at the lower doses.[38] As such, SSRIs should be tapered not in standard increments, such as by 25 mg each time, but rather as a proportion of the previous dose, such as 25%.[39] How quickly one tapers depends partly on how long they have been taking the medication and how high their dose currently is. While using a pill cutter or the liquid formulation is an option to taper, sometimes the taper plan is adjusted to match the available pill sizes. Skipping doses toward the end of a taper is recommended only for medications with a long half-life.

Keep in Mind: Discontinuation Symptoms

Some adolescents will stop their SSRI on their own or wean more quickly than the clinician recommended. This self-management can result in discontinuation symptoms and have a flu-like presentation with symptoms including headache, diarrhea, nausea, vomiting, dizziness, or fatigue. When seeing patients with these symptoms who are taking an SSRI, the clinician should inquire about their medication adherence. Discontinuation symptoms are more common from medications with short half-lives, such as sertraline.[38]

When to Refer

The clinician should consider referring the patient to a pediatric psychiatrist in the following circumstances:

- Anytime they are uncomfortable with the management of the patient's depression or comorbidities
- Depression in a preadolescent
- Significant interference with functioning, including symptoms that threaten the ability to achieve developmental goals (eg, attending school)
- Treatment resistance, or failure to improve after first-line medication
- Uncertain diagnosis
- Unusual medication side effects
- Polypharmacy complicating the treatment plan
- Multiple mental health comorbidities or a concern for mania or psychosis
- Depressive symptoms that are preceded by serious trauma (ie, abuse/neglect, child welfare involvement)

Most states now have a telephonic psychiatric consultative service or child psychiatry access program that can be used by primary care clinicians for consultation, care coordination, and/or education and training programs (www.nncpap.org). Clinicians should become familiar with state-based resources. Examples of these resources include

- Massachusetts Child Psychiatry Access Project
- Commonwealth of Pennsylvania Telephonic Psychiatric Consultation Service Program
- California Child and Adolescent Mental Health Access Portal
- Virginia Mental Health Access Program

Discharge and Referral Back to the Primary Care Clinician

Patients' depression may be successfully comanaged by psychiatrists and primary care clinicians. Once the patient's condition seems stable, the psychiatrist and pediatric clinician may determine that the primary management of depression will return to the pediatric clinician. Patients can be discharged when

- They are successfully weaned from the medication and there are no concerns for relapse.
- Their condition is stable with their medication and they need monitoring every 3 months for medication adherence, adverse effects, and depression symptom screening.
- If rating scales were used at baseline, repeated measures show significant decreases in total or subscale scores.

During the discharge process, discuss with the patient and their family the importance of ongoing monitoring of their mood and depressive symptoms. Depression relapses and recurrences are highly likely, especially when depression develops during adolescence.[36,40,41] After one depressive episode, approximately 50% to 60% of people will have at least one more depressive episode during their lifetime.[36,41] Specifically for adolescents, studies show that 30% to 70% will experience a relapse within 5 years of their first depressive episode.[36,41,42] Psychoeducation for patients and their caregivers is important so they can identify a relapse/recurrence, as well as use the behavioral activation strategies they have learned. It is critical that patients and families understand when and where they should seek help if there is a recurrence.

Lessons Learned About Depression and Depressive Disorder Management and Initial Treatment

Depression is common in adolescents, and management involves psychotherapy alone, a combination of psychotherapy and pharmacotherapy, and, sometimes also, a referral to a higher level of care.[6,8,9] Most adolescents will respond to this treatment approach, but treatment-resistant or relapsing cases warrant further diagnostic exploration and, often, comanagement with a psychiatrist.[35,41]

- Medication is only one part of the treatment plan. Encourage lifestyle modifications, mindfulness/grounding/relaxation techniques, and psychotherapy.
- CBT, IPT-A, DBT-A, and ACT are all types of evidence-based treatments best suited for depression.[11–13]
- Fluoxetine and escitalopram are most often used to treat moderate to severe depression and have FDA approval for this indication.[9,26,27,33]
- "Start low and go slow" with initiation of an SSRI.
- Review the black box warning for SSRIs with patients and families.
- Avoid polypharmacy if possible.
- Make one change at a time and use rating scales to monitor symptoms and treatment response.

Keywords: CBT, depression, escitalopram, fluoxetine, IPT-A, safety planning, suicide

Suggested Reading

Barber AE, Marass A. Universal depression screening for pediatric adolescent patients at well visits using the PHQ-9M within the pediatric primary care clinic. *J Dr Nurs Pract.* 2025:JDNP-2024–0035.R1 PMID: 40854675

Riddle MA, Campo JV. Group 1 medications for anxiety and depression. In: *Pediatric Psychopharmacology for Primary Care.* 4th ed. American Academy of Pediatrics; 2025:105–124

References

1. Weitzman C, Guevara J, Curtin M, Macias M; American Academy of Pediatrics Section on Developmental and Behavioral Pediatrics, Council on Early Childhood, and Committee on Psychosocial Aspects of Child and Family Health; Society for Developmental and Behavioral Pediatrics. Promoting optimal development: screening for mental health, emotional, and behavioral problems: clinical report. *Pediatrics*. 2025;156(3):e2025073172 PMID: 40850690
2. Foy JM, Green CM, Earls MF; American Academy of Pediatrics Committee on Psychosocial Aspects of Child and Family Health and Mental Health Leadership Work Group. Mental health competencies for pediatric practice. *Pediatrics*. 2019;144(5):e20192757 PMID: 31636143
3. Cunningham PJ. Beyond parity: primary care physicians' perspectives on access to mental health care. *Health Aff (Millwood)*. 2009;28(3):w490–w501 PMID: 19366722
4. Lee CM, Lutz J, Khau A, et al. Pediatric primary care perspectives of mental health services delivery during the COVID-19 pandemic. *Children (Basel)*. 2022;9(8):1186 PMID: 36010056
5. Gray GV, Brody DS, Hart MT. Primary care and the de facto mental health care system: improving care where it counts. *Manag Care Interface*. 2000;13(3):62–65 PMID: 11066279
6. Zuckerbrot RA, Cheung A, Jensen PS, Stein REK, Laraque D; GLAD-PC Steering Group. Guidelines for Adolescent Depression in Primary Care (GLAD-PC), I: practice preparation, identification, assessment, and initial management. *Pediatrics*. 2018;141(3):e20174081 PMID: 29483200
7. American Psychiatric Association. Depressive disorders. In: *Diagnostic and Statistical Manual of Mental Disorders*. 5th ed, text rev. American Psychiatric Association Publishing; 2022:177–214
8. Cheung AH, Zuckerbrot RA, Jensen PS, Laraque D, Stein REK; GLAD-PC Steering Group. Guidelines for Adolescent Depression in Primary Care (GLAD-PC), II: treatment and ongoing management. *Pediatrics*. 2018;141(3):e20174082 PMID: 29483201
9. March J, Silva S, Petrycki S, et al; Treatment for Adolescents With Depression Study (TADS) Team. Fluoxetine, cognitive-behavioral therapy, and their combination for adolescents with depression: Treatment for Adolescents With Depression Study (TADS) randomized controlled trial. *JAMA*. 2004;292(7):807–820 PMID: 15315995
10. March JS, Vitiello B. Clinical messages from the Treatment for Adolescents With Depression Study (TADS). *Am J Psychiatry*. 2009;166(10):1118–1123 PMID: 19723786
11. Weisz JR, McCarty CA, Valeri SM. Effects of psychotherapy for depression in children and adolescents: a meta-analysis. *Psychol Bull*. 2006;132(1):132–149 PMID: 16435960
12. David-Ferdon C, Kaslow NJ. Evidence-based psychosocial treatments for child and adolescent depression. *J Clin Child Adolesc Psychol*. 2008;37(1):62–104 PMID: 18444054
13. Zhou X, Hetrick SE, Cuijpers P, et al. Comparative efficacy and acceptability of psychotherapies for depression in children and adolescents: a systematic review and network meta-analysis. *World Psychiatry*. 2015;14(2):207–222 PMID: 26043339
14. Thielemann JFB, Kasparik B, König J, Unterhitzenberger J, Rosner R. A systematic review and meta-analysis of trauma-focused cognitive behavioral therapy for children and adolescents. *Child Abuse Negl*. 2022;134:105899 PMID: 36155943
15. Norcross JC, Wampold BE. Evidence-based therapy relationships: research conclusions and clinical practices. *Psychotherapy (Chic)*. 2011;48(1):98–102 PMID: 21401280
16. Wampold BE, Imel ZE. *The Great Psychotherapy Debate: The Evidence for What Makes Psychotherapy Work*. 2nd ed. Routledge; 2015

17. Lovato N, Gradisar M. A meta-analysis and model of the relationship between sleep and depression in adolescents: recommendations for future research and clinical practice. *Sleep Med Rev.* 2014;18(6):521–529 PMID: 24857255

18. Mohd Saat NZ, Hanawi SA, Hanafiah H, Ahmad M, Farah NMF, Abdul Rahman NAA. Relationship of screen time with anxiety, depression, and sleep quality among adolescents: a cross-sectional study. *Front Public Health.* 2024;12:1459952 PMID: 39678241

19. Munzer T, Parga-Belinkie J, Milkovich LM, et al; American Academy of Pediatrics Council on Communications and Media. Digital ecosystems, children, and adolescents. *Pediatrics.* 2026;157(2):e2025075320 PMID: 41556917

20. Riehm KE, Feder KA, Tormohlen KN, et al. Associations between time spent using social media and internalizing and externalizing problems among US youth. *JAMA Psychiatry.* 2019;76(12):1266–1273 PMID: 31509167

21. Eirich R, McArthur BA, Anhorn C, McGuinness C, Christakis DA, Madigan S. Association of screen time with internalizing and externalizing behavior problems in children 12 years or younger: a systematic review and meta-analysis. *JAMA Psychiatry.* 2022;79(5):393–405 PMID: 35293954

22. Teague S, Somoray K, Shatte A, et al. Digital media use and child health and development: a systematic review and meta-analysis. *JAMA Pediatr.* 2026;e260085 PMID: 41801211

23. Hilt LM, Swords CM, Webb CA. Randomized controlled trial of a mindfulness mobile application for ruminative adolescents. *J Clin Child Adolesc Psychol.* 2025;54(1):99–112 PMID: 36622879

24. D'Zurilla TJ, Nezu AM. Problem-solving therapy. In: Dobson KS, ed. *Handbook of Cognitive-Behavioral Therapies.* 3rd ed. Guilford Press; 2010:197–225

25. Bridge JA, Iyengar S, Salary CB, et al. Clinical response and risk for reported suicidal ideation and suicide attempts in pediatric antidepressant treatment: a meta-analysis of randomized controlled trials. *JAMA.* 2007;297(15):1683–1696 PMID: 17440145

26. Emslie GJ, Heiligenstein JH, Wagner KD, et al. Fluoxetine for acute treatment of depression in children and adolescents: a placebo-controlled, randomized clinical trial. *J Am Acad Child Adolesc Psychiatry.* 2002;41(10):1205–1215 PMID: 12364842

27. Wagner KD, Jonas J, Findling RL, Ventura D, Saikali K. A double-blind, randomized, placebo-controlled trial of escitalopram in the treatment of pediatric depression. *J Am Acad Child Adolesc Psychiatry.* 2006;45(3):280–288 PMID: 16540812

28. Walter HJ, Bukstein OG, Abright AR, et al. Clinical practice guideline for the assessment and treatment of children and adolescents with anxiety disorders. *J Am Acad Child Adolesc Psychiatry.* 2020;59(10):1107–1124 PMID: 32439401

29. Lexidrug. Fluoxetine: drug information. Retrieved March 21, 2026. https://online.lexi.com/lco/action/doc/retrieve/docid/chiphi_f/381212

30. Hemeryck A, Belpaire FM. Selective serotonin reuptake inhibitors and cytochrome P-450 mediated drug-drug interactions: an update. *Curr Drug Metab.* 2002;3(1):13–37 PMID: 11876575

31. Foong AL, Grindrod KA, Patel T, Kellar J. Demystifying serotonin syndrome (or serotonin toxicity). *Can Fam Physician.* 2018;64(10):720–727 PMID: 30315014

32. Simon LV, Torrico TJ, Keenaghan M. Serotonin syndrome. In: *StatPearls.* StatPearls Publishing; 2025. Updated March 2, 2024. Accessed February 20, 2026. https://www.ncbi.nlm.nih.gov/books/NBK482377

33. Emslie GJ, Ventura D, Korotzer A, Tourkodimitris S. Escitalopram in the treatment of adolescent depression: a randomized placebo-controlled multisite trial. *J Am Acad Child Adolesc Psychiatry.* 2009;48(7):721–729 PMID: 19465881

34. Yeh HH, Westphal J, Hu Y, et al. Diagnosed mental health conditions and risk of suicide mortality. *Psychiatr Serv.* 2019;70(9):750–757 PMID: 31185853

35. Emslie GJ, Mayes T, Porta G, et al. Treatment of Resistant Depression in Adolescents (TORDIA): week 24 outcomes. *Am J Psychiatry.* 2010;167(7):782–791 PMID: 20478877

36. Desai Boström AE, Cars T, Hellner C, Lundberg J. Recovery and recurrence from major depression in adolescence and adulthood. *Acta Psychiatr Scand.* 2025;151(5):625–633 PMID: 39756801

37. Children's Hospital of Philadelphia. Treatment of non-responders or resistant depression. Accessed April 19, 2026. https://www.chop.edu/clinical-pathway/risk-diagnosis-depression-treatment-non-responders-or-resistant-depression

38. Sørensen A, Juhl Jørgensen K, Munkholm K. Clinical practice guideline recommendations on tapering and discontinuing antidepressants for depression: a systematic review. *Ther Adv Psychopharmacol.* 2022;12:20451253211067656 PMID: 35173954

39. Horowitz MA, Taylor D. Tapering of SSRI treatment to mitigate withdrawal symptoms. *Lancet Psychiatry.* 2019;6(6):538–546 PMID: 30850328

40. Kovacs M, Feinberg TL, Crouse-Novak M, Paulauskas SL, Pollock M, Finkelstein R. Depressive disorders in childhood, II: a longitudinal study of the risk for a subsequent major depression. *Arch Gen Psychiatry.* 1984;41(7):643–649 PMID: 673242

41. Kennard BD, Emslie GJ, Mayes TL, Hughes JL. Relapse and recurrence in pediatric depression. *Child Adolesc Psychiatr Clin N Am.* 2006;15(4):1057–1079, xi PMID: 16952775

42. McCauley E, Myers K, Mitchell J, Calderon R, Schloredt K, Treder R. Depression in young people: initial presentation and clinical course. *J Am Acad Child Adolesc Psychiatry.* 1993;32(4):714–722 PMID: 8340290

CHAPTER 12

Attention-Deficit/ Hyperactivity Disorder

Treatment of patients with subthreshold attention and hyperactivity symptoms and attention-deficit/hyperactivity disorder (ADHD) can be initiated in the pediatric primary care setting. The American Academy of Pediatrics endorses that to promote the optimal development of children, behavioral and emotional screening should happen routinely in pediatric primary care so early intervention can occur.[1] Treatment may include parent training, school-based interventions, psychotherapy, and/or medication management, depending on age and severity of ADHD.[2] Pediatric clinicians are well positioned to address the behavioral and mental health of their patients because of their longitudinal relationships with patients and their families, whole-child approach, and ability to initiate treatment and/or serve as bridge to mental health specialists.[3]

Screening for and diagnostic assessment of ADHD were discussed in Chapters 7, Irritable Mood, and 8, Attention-Deficit/Hyperactivity Disorder and Learning Difficulties. Some cases presented subthreshold ADHD symptoms that caused impairment in functioning but did not rise to the level of a clinical diagnosis, while others met criteria for a diagnosable disorder and required a higher level of clinical and medical intervention. It is important to understand the difference between the two to find the best avenue for care and management in the clinical setting. Attention issues, hyperactivity, and executive functioning challenges can all be normal parts of child development, especially in early childhood, and should not always be pathologized but used as context clues to understand how these symptoms interfere with functioning; thus, helping patients distinguish between managing symptoms and managing a disorder is an important distinction. While diagnostic criteria for ADHD will be reviewed, the purpose of this chapter is to review psychoeducation, psychotherapy, medication management, referral to psychologists and/or psychiatrists, and the comanagement of patients with ADHD.

When discussing treatment options for ADHD with a patient, it is important to provide them with psychoeducation about ADHD, including its impact on functioning; evidence-based treatment options; medication options (if applicable); and brief interventions to help maintain and stabilize the patient's mood and functioning as best as possible within one's role as the primary care clinician.

Keep in Mind: A Primary Care Clinician's Role

- Facilitate brief interventions in the office, including evidence-based screening tools.
- Initiate first-line medications as clinically indicated.
- Provide referrals to mental health specialists.
- Provide supportive monitoring until a mental health specialist is involved and the patient's condition is stable with medication.

Because aggression and disruptive behavior can be a symptom of ADHD and many of its coexisting conditions, aggression can both mimic ADHD symptoms and improve with ADHD treatment, thus complicating ADHD monitoring and treatment. As such, aggression is also discussed in this chapter.

Review the Diagnostic Criteria for ADHD

Attention-deficit/hyperactivity disorder is diagnosed when there is a persistent pattern of inattention and/or hyperactivity/impulsivity that interferes with functioning or development.[4,5] Symptoms should be present for at least 6 months and occur in 2 settings (home and school, typically), and some symptoms should be present before 12 years of age.[4,5]

Symptoms of inattention may include[2,4–6]

- Mistakes on typically automatic or quick tasks
- Not following directions
- Difficulty with organization
- Easily distracted

Symptoms of hyperactivity/impulsivity may include[2,4–6]

- Fidgeting
- Difficulty staying seated or waiting in line
- Always on the go
- Blurting out answers
- Trouble taking turns

There are 3 subtypes of ADHD.[2,4–6]

- Combined subtype
- Predominately inattentive subtype
- Predominantly hyperactive/impulsive subtype

Additional points to consider include

- When scoring the NICHQ Vanderbilt Assessment Scale, the clinician will note that 6 symptoms are needed for each subtype and must be causing impairment in more than 1 setting to meet the *Diagnostic and Statistical Manual of Mental Disorders, Fifth Edition, Text Revision* criteria for ADHD.[4,6]
- The symptoms cannot be better explained by another mental health disorder (eg, mood disorder, anxiety disorder, substance use disorder [SUD]).[4,5]

A helpful clinical pathway for the evaluation and treatment of ADHD can be found online (www.chop.edu/clinical-pathway/adhd-clinical-pathway).

Psychoeducation

When discussing ADHD with patients and caregivers, it can be helpful to explain that ADHD is a neurodevelopmental disorder. According to the World Health Organization *International Classification of Diseases, 11th Revision*, a neurodevelopmental disorder is characterized by differences in and the developmental trajectory of the acquisition and execution of specific cognitive, behavioral, and social functioning.[5] Attention-deficit/hyperactivity disorder is a neurodevelopmental disorder; other neurodevelopmental disorders include autism spectrum disorder and intellectual developmental disorders.[4,5] It is estimated to affect approximately 11% of children and adolescents in the United States between the ages of 3 and 17 years, with a 3:1 ratio of male to female prevalence.[7–10] Attention-deficit/hyperactivity disorder can affect not only a child's ability to regulate behavior, focus, and control emotions but also their peer relationships, their relationships with their caregivers and teachers, their school performance, and other activities, such as sports or hobbies. It is important to help caregivers understand that ADHD is not an intellectual disability, nor is it related to intelligence or cognitive functioning. It can, however, make aspects of daily life challenging, including academic functioning, social skills, and behavior management.[5,11] Caregivers should learn how to manage components of inattention, hyperactivity, and impulsivity and their impact on daily functioning.

➤ What should clinicians say to a caregiver who states, "He's just like me when I was a kid, and I turned out fine."

First, praise them for sharing their childhood experiences. Next, explain that leading research indicates that ADHD has a genetic component, meaning that ADHD (or attention-deficit disorder, or hyperactivity disorder) tends to run in families.[4,12] It can be helpful for the caregiver to recognize that the goal of diagnosing and treating ADHD is to spare their child any distress that the caregiver may have experienced because of their symptoms as a child.[12] Then, discuss the rating scales that can be used to compare their child's behavior to that of their same-aged peers.[6] Although other children may act similarly (eg, all children have difficulty paying attention or waiting their turn), it is about how their child's behavior interferes with their child's functioning that concerns pediatric clinicians.[11] Last, explain how common ADHD is and decrease any stigma around treatment.[7,8]

➤ What should clinicians say when a caregiver states, "I don't want to label them"?

Children with ADHD are often already labeled by their teachers or peers as "lazy" or "bad" without an understanding of the underlying neurodevelopmental challenges driving their behavior. Helping change that label to "ADHD" allows others to understand why the child has these behaviors and helps them receive the appropriate supports and educational services.[11] It can be helpful to provide families with meaningful examples or analogies, such as imagining that a child has diabetes. Because diabetes is a serious medical condition, it would be imperative to let caregivers and schools know about this medical diagnosis to enhance collaborative care and shared decision-making and to reduce fear of stigma. Mental health diagnoses should be treated with the same lens as chronic medical conditions. Additionally, using diagnostic labels allows for greater access to psychosocial and school-based services.

Resources

Books

- *The Explosive Child: A New Approach for Understanding and Parenting Easily Frustrated, Chronically Inflexible Children*, 6th Edition, by Ross W. Greene, PhD
- *The Gift of ADHD: How to Transform Your Child's Problems Into Strengths*, 2nd Edition, by Lara Honos-Webb, PhD
- *How to Talk So Kids Will Listen and Listen So Kids Will Talk* by Adele Faber and Elaine Mazlish
- *Smart but Scattered: The Revolutionary Executive Skills Approach to Helping Kids Reach Their Potential*, 2nd Edition, by Peg Dawson, EdD; Richard Guare, PhD; and Colin Guare, MS

- *Taking Charge of ADHD: The Complete Authoritative Guide for Parents*, 4th Edition, by Russell A. Barkley, PhD
- *Thriving With ADHD: The Ultimate Guide for Parents of Children With ADHD* by Michael Marsden

Websites

- American Academy of Child and Adolescent Psychiatry—ADHD Resource Center (www.aacap.org/aacap/Families_and_Youth/Resource_Centers/ADHD_Resource_Center/Home.aspx)
- Centers for Disease Control and Prevention—Attention-Deficit/Hyperactivity Disorder (www.cdc.gov/adhd)
- Children and Adults with Attention-Deficit/Hyperactivity Disorder (https://chadd.org)
- Child Mind Institute (https://childmind.org)
- HealthyChildren.org—ADHD (www.healthychildren.org/English/health-issues/conditions/adhd/Pages/default.aspx)

Evidence-Based Treatment Options

The Multimodal Treatment of Children With ADHD (MTA) study was a multisite study to evaluate treatments of ADHD including behavioral therapy, medications, and a combination of the two.[16] This study is important because it was the first time the safety and relative effectiveness of 2 treatments (alone and in combination) were studied for a period as long as 14 months and compared to routine care. The results were published in 1999 and showed that

- Combination treatment (eg, behavioral therapy and medication management) and medication management alone were significantly better than behavioral treatment alone.[16]
- The benefits of treatment lasted 14 months but were not sustained in the long term at the 2- and 3-year follow-ups, likely due to medications being discontinued by the patients.[17]
- Combination treatment also improved social functioning and parent-child relationships, whereas either treatment alone did not.[17]
- Combination treatment resulted in lower doses of medication than if medication was used alone.[16]

In practice, the treatment approach for patients with ADHD depends on a patient's age and severity of symptoms (**Box 12-1**).

Box 12-1. Attention-Deficit/Hyperactivity Disorder Management by Severity[a,b]

- **Mild:** psychotherapy, consideration of medication alone
- **Moderate:** psychotherapy + recommendation of pharmacotherapy medication[c]
- **Severe:** psychotherapy + pharmacotherapy medication + consideration of referral to a specialist

[a] Wolraich ML, Hagan JF Jr, Allan C, et al; American Academy of Pediatrics Subcommittee on Children and Adolescents With Attention-Deficit/Hyperactivity Disorder. Clinical practice guideline for the diagnosis, evaluation, and treatment of attention-deficit/hyperactivity disorder in children and adolescents. *Pediatrics.* 2019;144(4):e20192528.

[b] MTA Cooperative Group. A 14-month randomized clinical trial of treatment strategies for attention-deficit/hyperactivity disorder. *Arch Gen Psychiatry.* 1999;56(12):1073–1086.

[c] For children 3–5 years old, pharmacotherapy medication is recommended only for severe cases and the first-line of treatment is Behavioral Parent Training.

Special Populations to Consider

Two age demographics warrant special treatment consideration: preschoolers and adolescents.[18] These groups (ie, children between 3 and 5 years of age and 12 years and older) are considered to have "complex ADHD." The diagnosis of ADHD in these groups should be done by a clinician with specialized training or expertise (eg, psychiatrist, developmental behavioral pediatrician, child neurologist, and pediatric providers with advanced training) and should be comprehensive to exclude other diagnoses or incorporate coexisting conditions into the treatment plan. Although treatment guidelines exist, research is limited, so shared decision-making with patients/families is important.[19]

Evidence-based interventions (eg, BPT for preschool-aged children and organizational skills training for adolescents) targeted at impairments across settings are a mainstay of treatment for all children and adolescents with ADHD.[19] In preschool-aged children, medications are typically used only in patients with severe symptoms. Keep in mind that preschool-aged children may experience more medication adverse effects, including irritability, loss of appetite, and sleep disturbance.[20,21] Consultation with a developmental and behavioral pediatrician may be necessary for medication management. For adolescents, medication management should include careful assessment for coexisting conditions, such as anxiety, depression, and SUD, as well as social risk factors, such as poverty, so that the treatment plan can address all contributors to symptoms.

Although ADHD is often thought of as a childhood disorder that primarily interferes with functioning at school, it is a neurodevelopmental disorder that can have impacts across the lifespan. Therefore, special care should be taken in helping adolescent patients transition to adult care so that there are no lapses in treatment plans during transition.

Psychotherapy

There are specific evidence-based therapies recommended for use with children with ADHD and their families.[22] Refer to these therapies by name when discussing them with the patient and family because not all psychotherapy modalities have been shown to be effective in the treatment and management of ADHD.

- Behavioral therapy: Specifically Behavior Parent Training (BPT), Parent Management Training (PMT), Family Behavioral Therapy (FBT), and Parent-Child Interaction Therapy (PCIT). Cognitive behavioral therapy (CBT) can also be used with older children.[11,13,14]
- Social skills training.[11,22]
- Organizational skills training.[11,22]

➤ How do I incorporate behavioral strategies into a busy practice?

Behavioral treatment of ADHD stems from treatment related to disruptive behavior disorders, such as Behavioral Parent Training (BPT) or Parent-Child Interaction Therapy (PCIT).[13,14] Here are a few strategies you can incorporate into your practice.

- The importance of praise: Children with ADHD often receive a lot of corrective feedback that can be easily perceived by the child as negative or punishment, because impulsive behavior can lead to frequent mistakes. It's important to help parents balance this by intentionally noticing what their child is doing well and providing praise. Praise can be simple and nonverbal, such as offering a smile, hug, or high five, or specific and spoken, such as commenting on a calm request or a thoughtful choice. A useful guideline is to offer positive feedback far more often than corrections, aiming for roughly 4 praises for every 1 critique.[11,15]
- Positive reinforcement: Similarly, positive reinforcement uses strategies such as praise and rewards for positive behavior. It is one of the most powerful methods parents can use to improve their child's behavior. The goal is to increase the likelihood that the behavior will occur in the future.
  — "Catch your child being good": Just as the name implies, this can be a tool for parents to be on the lookout for specific things their child does well and provide labeled praise.[7] For example, "Great job putting your plate into the sink" or "I like how you helped your sister clean up."
- Home-school collaboration: Parents need to align with teachers in a manner that suggests they are "all on the same team," as a strong parent-teacher relationship can be crucial for enhancing the learning environment and recognizing areas for growth.[11]
- Organization help: Children with ADHD tend to have difficulties with executive functioning, including the ability to plan, organize, initiate, monitor, and adapt behavior in novel or complex situations. Children with ADHD can be disorganized, and this can affect their performance at school and at home.[11] Parents and teachers can often misattribute disorganization to laziness rather than differences in the brains of children with ADHD. These differences in executive function are best met with a calm adult who helps provide structure and organization. There are types of therapy interventions known as organizational skills training that specifically address these areas.

••• Communication Pearl ••• Psychotherapy

A key component in psychotherapy for ADHD involves family-based approaches. Caregivers can learn skills to help improve communication and organization, reduce family conflict, and support emotion regulation. Home-school collaboration is also key. It's important to help caregivers understand the role of advocate and collaborator when it comes to supporting a child with ADHD through their educational journey.[11]

Pharmacotherapy

Pharmacotherapy should be considered for patients with moderate to severe ADHD and can be initiated by a pediatric clinician. There are several classes of US Food and Drug Administration (FDA)–approved medications for the treatment of ADHD, including stimulants (methylphenidate and amphetamine), α_2-adrenergic agonists (guanfacine and clonidine), and one of the selective norepinephrine reuptake inhibitors (atomoxetine).[2,23,24] Although some preparations of methylphenidate and amphetamine (immediate-release Adderall) are approved down to age 3 years, in general ADHD medication FDA approval is for children 6 years and older.[2] Preschool-aged children are more likely to have side effects, including mood lability and dysphoria, from stimulants.[2] Use of methylphenidate in children younger than 6 years requires informed consent.

Keep in Mind: Psychopharmacology[2,23,25]

- Methylphenidate: blocks dopamine uptake by inhibiting dopamine transporter (DAT) and norepinephrine transporter (NET), which increases dopamine and norepinephrine levels
- Amphetamine: blocks DAT and NET but also increases catecholamine release, which produces a more potent increase in dopamine and norepinephrine levels than methylphenidate
- Guanfacine or clonidine: stimulates α_{2A}-adrenergic receptors in the prefrontal cortex, which increases signal transmission in the prefrontal cortex
- Atomoxetine: blocks reuptake at noradrenergic neurons (NET), which increases norepinephrine levels and may indirectly increase dopamine levels in the prefrontal cortex

Commonly Prescribed ADHD Medications

Clinicians should be familiar with the most commonly prescribed ADHD medications in each class (stimulants, α_2-adrenergic agonists, and selective norepinephrine reuptake inhibitor), including any potential adverse effects and guidance for monitoring.

Stimulants

- Immediate-release stimulants: start to take effect in 20 to 30 minutes and, depending on the drug and formulation, reach peak in 1 to 3 hours before wearing off in 4 to 6 hours[23,25]
  - Most common adverse effects: headache, stomachache, sleep disturbance, loss of appetite[2,25,26]
  - Uncommon but potentially serious adverse effects: priapism, psychosis[2,25,26]
  - Monitoring parameters: weight, height, blood pressure, pulse
    - Methylphenidate hydrochloride (eg, Methylin, Ritalin)
      - Available as oral solution, chewable, or crushable tablet
    - Dexmethylphenidate (eg, Focalin)
      - Available in crushable tablet
    - Dextroamphetamine (eg, ProCentra)
      - Available as oral solution
    - Amphetamine sulfate (eg, Evekeo)
      - Oral disintegrating tablet or crushable tablet
    - Amphetamine-dextroamphetamine (eg, Adderall)
      - Available in crushable tablet
    - Dextroamphetamine sulfate (eg, Zenzedi)
      - Available in crushable tablet
- Extended-release stimulants: start to take effect within 30 to 45 minutes and, depending on the drug and formulation, reach a peak in 2 to 4 hours before wearing off in 8 to 12 hours[2,23,24]
  - Most common adverse effects: headache, stomachache, sleep disturbance, loss of appetite[2,25,26]
  - Uncommon but potentially serious adverse effects: priapism, psychosis[2,25,26]
  - Monitoring parameters: weight, height, blood pressure, pulse
    - Methylphenidate (eg, Concerta)
      - Must be swallowed whole
      - Immediately releases 22% and then slowly releases 78%
    - Methylphenidate (eg, Focalin XR)
      - Can be opened and sprinkled
      - Contains 50% immediate-release beads and 50% enteric-coated, delayed-release beads
    - Amphetamine (eg, Adderall XR)
      - Can be opened and sprinkled
      - Immediately releases 50% and then slowly releases 50%
    - Lisdexamfetamine (eg, Vyvanse)
      - Capsule can be opened and sprinkled or tablet can be chewed.
      - Prodrug, so it can take longer to take effect (1 hour) and last longer (13–14 hours).

α_2-Adrenergic Agonists

- Second-line, but may be a good choice when there are ADHD and tic disorders, sleep problems, autism spectrum disorder, and/or aggression[2,23,24]; sedative effects within 1 to 2 hours, but may take 2 to 3 weeks before any behavioral changes are noted and 4 to 6 weeks for full effect[2,27]
  - Potential adverse effects: somnolence, dry mouth, headache, nausea, hypotension, constipation[2,23,25]
  - Monitoring parameters: pulse, blood pressure
    - Guanfacine (eg, Intuniv, guanfacine immediate-release)
      - Specific to the α_{2A}-receptor subtype, which means it targets attention and executive function.
      - Immediate release starts to take effect in 1 to 2 hours, peaks at 1 to 4 hours, but may not wear off for 24 hours.
      - This is indicated for hypertension and used off-label for ADHD.[28]
      - Extended release (Intuniv) reaches peak in 5 hours and remains steady over 24 hours.
    - Clonidine (eg, Catapres, Kapvay)
      - Nonspecifically interacts with α_{2A}-, α_{2B}-, and α_{2C}-receptor subtypes, which means it may be more likely to produce side effects related to sedation, hypotension, or bradycardia
      - Starts to take effect in 30 to 60 minutes, reaches a peak in 2 to 4 hours (immediate release) or 4 to 7 hours (extended release), and wears off after 8 hours[29]

Selective Norepinephrine Reuptake Inhibitor

- Second-line, but may be a good choice when there is coexisting anxiety or a contraindication to stimulant use[2,23,24]; may see some effect sooner, but can take 4 to 6 weeks to reach full effect[2]
  - Potential adverse effects: nausea, loss of appetite, weight loss, dizziness[2,23]
  - Monitoring parameters: weight, height, pulse, suicidal ideation
    - Atomoxetine (eg, Strattera)
      - US Food and Drug Administration black box warning about increased risk for suicidal thoughts and behaviors

For more detailed information on FDA-approved ADHD medications, a useful resource is available online (www.adhdmedicationguide.com).

••• Communication Pearl •••
Genetic Testing

Some caregivers may ask if genetic testing is an option to determine the best medication for their child. Because of the large number of medication options and extensive variability in patient responses to any drug, genetic testing is of particular interest. However, there is not currently enough evidence to support pharmacogenetic testing in clinical care.[23,24]

First-Line Treatment: Stimulants

Stimulants are considered the first-line treatment and are highly effective, with approximately 70% of patients responding to the first trial and 90% after a second trial.[25] If the first medication does not achieve desired results in the patient, try a different class before using a non-stimulant.[2,23] Refer to **Table 12–1** for dosage information for commonly prescribed stimulant medications in children older than 6 years. A helpful online resource about medications to treat ADHD can be found online (www.chop.edu/clinical-pathway/adhd-medications).

Table 12–1. Commonly Used Stimulant Medications in Children Older Than 6 Years[a–d]

Stimulant Medication	Initial Dosage	Titration	Max Dosage
Methylphenidate regular-release	3–6 years: 1.25 mg per dose twice daily 6 years and older: 0.3 mg/kg per dose or 2.5–5 mg per dose	3–6 years: Titrate to effect weekly (typical dose is 3.75–30 mg/day in 2–3 divided doses). 6 years and older: 0.1 mg/kg per dose or 5–10 mg/day at weekly intervals (typical dose is 0.3–1 mg/kg/day).	2 mg/kg/ day or 60 mg/day
Methylphenidate extended-release capsules (Metadate CD, Ritalin LA)	6 years and older: 20 mg/day	10–20 mg/day at weekly intervals	60 mg/day
Methylphenidate osmotic controlled-release tablets (Concerta)	6 years and older: 18 mg/day (Initial dose may be higher for children and adolescents already using methylphenidate.)	10–20 mg/day at weekly intervals	60 mg/day
Dexmethylphenidate immediate-release (Focalin)	6 years and older: 2.5 mg twice daily	2.5–5 mg/day at weekly intervals until optimal response obtained	20 mg/day
Dexmethylphenidate extended-release (Focalin XR)	5 mg/day	5 mg/day at weekly intervals until optimal response obtained	30 mg/day

Continued on the next page

Table 12–1 (*continued*)

Stimulant Medication	Initial Dosage	Titration	Max Dosage
Amphetamine-dextroamphetamine (Adderall)	3–5 years: 2.5 mg/day 6 years and older: 5 mg once or twice daily	3–5 years: 2.5 mg at weekly intervals until optimal response obtained 6 years and older: 5 mg at weekly intervals until optimal response obtained	40 mg/day in 1–3 divided doses
Amphetamine-dextroamphetamine (Adderall XR)	6–12 years: 5–10 mg/day 13–17 years: 10 mg/day	5–10 mg/day at weekly intervals until optimal response obtained. 13–17 years: Increase to 20 mg/day after 1 week if symptoms are not controlled.	30 mg/day
Lisdexamfetamine (Vyvanse)	6 years and older: 20–30 mg/day	10–20 mg/day at 3–7 day intervals until optimal response obtained at lowest effective dose	70 mg/day

Abbreviations: max, maximum.

[a] Lexidrug. Methylphenidate: drug information. Retrieved March 27, 2026. https://online.lexi.com.

[b] Lexidrug. Dexmethylphenidate: drug information. Retrieved March 27, 2026. https://online.lexi.com.

[c] Lexidrug. Amphetamine/dextroamphetamine (Adderall): drug information. Retrieved March 27, 2026. https://online.lexi.com.

[d] Lexidrug. Lisdexamfetamine (Vyvanse): drug information. Retrieved March 27, 2026. https://online.lexi.com.

Safety of Stimulants

Stimulants have been on the market for more than 50 years and are FDA approved for the treatment of ADHD.[23,24] The MTA study was a large randomized controlled trial with years of observational follow-up.[16,17] There is a low risk of overdose harm from stimulants. However, the possible risks of stimulants include[2,25,26]

- Drug dependence and misuse potential
  - No reports of dependence developing in children using therapeutic doses.
  - Children with ADHD who are treated with stimulants are not more likely than those who did not receive stimulants to have substance misuse later in life, and some studies demonstrate a lower risk for SUD in children who are treated with stimulants.[19]
  - A black box warning on methylphenidate, dexmethylphenidate, and amphetamine package inserts warns that these medications should not be used in patients with recent stimulant drug abuse or dependence.[25] These medications are still recommended for ADHD treatment in adolescents who use nicotine, alcohol, or opioids, although they should be monitored for signs of stimulant misuse.

  - Diversion and misuse can be an issue with adolescents, and prevention should include education and close monitoring, including using a state prescription drug monitoring program to track prescription dates. Immediate-release formulations should not be used if a concern for possible diversion exists, as these are easier to misuse. For this reason, extended-release methylphenidate is often preferred for adolescents, including college students.[19,25]
- Growth deceleration
  - On average, less than 2 cm over 3 years. Studies are inconsistent and report anywhere from a 2- to 4-cm impact on adult height, but some studies do not demonstrate any impact.[16,20] Monitoring of height and weight is recommended and faltering can be managed with medication "holidays," increased caloric intake, or referral to a specialist for further evaluation and treatment.
- Serious cardiovascular events
  - Generally only in patients with known cardiac disease, so family history and screening before initiation are important. Ongoing screening questions periodically during treatment are recommended.
- Increase in blood pressure
  - Generally not clinically significant, but blood pressure should be checked at follow-up visits.
- Exacerbation of tics
  - Likely unmasks a tic disorder rather than causes it.
- Priapism
  - Only methylphenidate preparations.

Keep in Mind: Stimulant Prescribing Rules[2,26]

Stimulants are Schedule II controlled substances under the Drug Enforcement Administration because they pose a high risk of abuse and dependence. Stimulants have a black box warning, which highlights both the cardiovascular risk and the risk for misuse, abuse, and dependence, which the clinician should discuss with patients and families. Follow state laws about what regulations clinicians should follow, but in general

- Give only a 30-day supply at one time. If giving refills, they should specify a future fill date.
- Send the prescription electronically.
- Review risk for misuse/diversion with the patient and family, including safe medication storage.
- Check the prescription drug monitoring program database to monitor for duplicate prescriptions.

Contraindications for Stimulants

Stimulants should be used with caution or avoided in patients with the following conditions.[2,26] If a patient has a history of any of these, it is recommended that the clinician consult with a specialist in that area before prescribing a stimulant medication.

- Severe cardiovascular disease
- Psychosis
- Severe anxiety/agitation
- Glaucoma
- Liver disease
- Drug dependence
- Seizure disorder not yet stabilized on anticonvulsants
- Patients taking monoamine oxidate inhibitors and St John's wort

Screening for Cardiac Risks

Before prescribing a patient a stimulant medication for ADHD, screen for cardiac disease and review a thorough cardiac family history. Only children with risk factors need to undergo electrocardiography before medication initiation.[2,26] Stimulant medications can be used in children with congenital heart disease, but the patient's cardiologist should be included in the discussion about the pros and cons of starting a stimulant medication.

Personal risk factors include[2,26]

- Syncope
- Chest pain with exercise
- Exercise intolerance
- Irregular heart rate

Family risk factors include[2,26]

- Sudden death before the age of 50 years
- Wolff-Parkinson-White syndrome
- Long QT syndrome
- Hypertrophic cardiomyopathy
- Marfan syndrome

Keep in Mind: Stimulants and Personality[30]

A small proportion of patients will report feeling like a zombie or an NPC (non-player character) in a video game. This is most often related to the dosage and will resolve with an adjusted lower dose or alternative stimulant formulation. At the appropriate dosage, a child should feel more focused and less impulsive. Some children describe it as turning down the volume on background noise so they can focus on their teacher/caregiver better. Children taking ADHD medications can be just as creative and joyful as those whose ADHD is untreated. Adolescents should participate in their treatment plan and may develop insight into when they need to take their stimulant, such as a school day, and when they may take a medication holiday, such as during a vacation.

Monitoring for Adverse Effects

While there are possible adverse effects of each stimulant medication, some occur more often than others. Counsel patients taking stimulant medications about possible appetite suppression, headache, stomachache, and insomnia.

To minimize adverse effects, do not increase the dose to increase duration if already experiencing side effects. Instead, choose a longer-acting medication or add a short-acting stimulant midday.

Keep in Mind: Attention-Deficit/Hyperactivity Disorder Medications and Differences by Sex

Girls are less likely to be diagnosed and treated for ADHD. When they do start medication, it is often at an older age than boys.[7,8] There are a few possible theories as to why this happens.[7,8]

- Under-detection: Girls may exhibit less disruptive behavior, as they have more inattention than hyperactivity symptoms.
- Diagnostic overshadowing: Girls are more likely to be treated for anxiety or depression before receiving ADHD treatment.
- Diagnostic bias: Pediatric researchers have learned that boys are more likely to have ADHD based on historical precedence.

It is important to be aware of when bias, including sociocultural norms, may be contributing to the overdiagnosis/underdiagnosis and treatment of ADHD.

➤ What if a patient reports decreased appetite while taking their stimulant?

- Recommend that the patient take their medication after eating breakfast.
- The caregiver can increase calories at dinner or allow a "double dinner" by offering a second meal instead of a lower-calorie snack after school.
- When the patient is not hungry at lunch, they can be offered something to drink that is high calorie, such as a smoothie or high protein milk.
- The caregiver can give the patient medication holidays on days when not in school, depending on the individual patient and family.
- Consider cyproheptadine (off-label).
- The patient can switch to a shorter-acting medication and be given a second dose after lunch.
- The family can wait it out: while decreased appetite is common, it is often worse in the first year of taking the medication.

➤ What if a patient reports sleep disruption while taking their stimulant?

- Educate on sleep hygiene: Set a consistent bedtime; have a calming bedtime routine; remove screens from the bedroom; provide a dark, cool bedroom; and no naps before bedtime.
- If the patient is taking a long-acting medication, ensure that the dose is taken at least 12 hours before bedtime. Consider a shorter-acting medication if necessary.
- Consider adding another medication, such as melatonin (not FDA approved) or clonidine (off-label).

Second-Line Treatment: Selective Norepinephrine Reuptake Inhibitor

Non-stimulants, such as atomoxetine, are generally used when a patient does not respond to 2 stimulants, has intolerable side effects of a stimulant, or there is a contraindication to stimulant use. Since 90% of patients will have a beneficial response to one of the stimulants, it is recommended to try at least 2 classes of stimulants before switching to a non-stimulant.[16] Atomoxetine may be considered first line when an adolescent has a history of stimulant misuse or abuse.[19] Atomoxetine (Strattera) is the only selective norepinephrine reuptake inhibitor with FDA approval in children aged 6 years and older (Table 12-2).

Table 12-2. Selective Norepinephrine Reuptake Inhibitor for ADHD Treatment[a]

Medication	Initial Dosage	Titration	Max Dosage
Atomoxetine (Strattera)	≤70 kg: 0.5 mg/kg/day >70 kg: 40 mg/day	≤70 kg: after a minimum of 3 days, increase to 1.2 mg/kg/day; once or twice daily. >70 kg: after a minimum of 3 days, increase to 80 mg/day; administer once or divide into 2 doses; may increase if needed to 100 mg/day in 2–4 additional weeks.	1.4 mg/kg/day or 100 mg/day, whichever is less. Doses >1.2 mg/kg/day have not shown additional benefit.

Abbreviation: max, maximum.

[a] Lexidrug. Atomoxetine (Strattera): drug information. Retrieved March 27, 2026. https://online.lexi.com.

Aggressive Behavior in Children and Adolescents

In children and adolescents with ADHD, impulsivity can lead to aggression. They can have a low frustration tolerance, which leads to emotional and behavioral dysregulation. Treating ADHD symptoms can help with behavioral outbursts, so for children with aggressive behavior, first consider if their ADHD is being appropriately treated.[16,17]

Attention-deficit/hyperactivity disorder can coexist with other mental health conditions in which aggression is a prominent symptom, including autism, SUD, bipolar disorder, psychosis, and conduct disorder.[2,4]

- Is the aggression impulsive? Strongly consider ADHD.
- Is the aggression emotional? Consider ADHD, mood disorder, or substance use.
- Is the aggression anxious? Consider anxiety or trauma.
- Is the aggression disorganized or nonlogical? Consider psychosis, bipolar disorder, or substance use.
- Is the aggression premeditated? Consider conduct disorder.

If the patient's aggression is suspected to be ADHD related, the timing of when the patient displays aggression during the day may help determine the etiology.

- During school
  - Could it be stimulant related?
    - Withhold the stimulant for a week to see if symptoms continue or resolve.
      - If symptoms resolve, consider decreasing the dose or switching to another class of medication.
      - If symptoms continue, consider behavioral and/or school-based interventions and restart the stimulant.
  - School-related triggers
    - Is there a specific class where this is an issue?
    - Any social factors, such as bullying?
    - Learning difficulty?
    - Anxiety?
- After school or in the afternoon
  - Could this be due to the stimulant wearing off?
    - Often short-lived and does not require intervention, but if severe, can treat with an immediate-release stimulant to help taper dose gradually.
    - Use behavioral interventions.

- All day
  - Consider trauma as a possible etiology.
  - Consider titrating the stimulant dose up or switching classes of medication.
  - If the dose is already maximized or the patient did not respond to 2 stimulant medications, consider adding an α_2-adrenergic agonist (**Table 12-3**).

Table 12–3. α_2-Adrenergic Agonists[a,b]

Medication	Initial Dosage	Titration	Max Dosage
Guanfacine IR	5 years and older and ≤25 kg: 0.25 mg once daily 5 years and older and >25 kg: 0.5 mg/day	0.25 mg every 3–4 days 5 years and older and >25 kg: 0.5 mg every 3–4 days	3 mg/day divided 2–3 times per day 5 years and older and >25 kg: 4 mg/day divided 2–3 times per day
Guanfacine ER (Intuniv)	5 years and older and ≤25 kg: 1 mg/day 5 years and older and >25 kg: 1 mg/day	5 years and older and ≤25 kg: 1 mg every 2 weeks 5 years and older and >25 kg: 1 mg at weekly intervals to a target dose range of 0.05–0.12 mg/kg/day	5 years and older and <25 kg: 3 mg/day 5–12 years and >25 kg: 4 mg/day 13 years and older: 7 mg/day (monotherapy) or 4 mg/day (adjunct with other stimulants)
Clonidine IR	≤45 kg: 0.05 mg (50 mcg) at bedtime >45 kg: 0.1 mg (100 mcg) at bedtime	≤45 kg: 0.05 mg/day every 3–7 days; increments given as 0.05 mg (50 mcg) twice daily, then 3 times daily, then 4 times daily >45 kg: 0.1 mg/day (100 mcg/day) every 3–7 days; increments given as twice daily, then 3 times daily, then 4 times daily	27–40.5 kg: 0.2 mg/day (200 mcg/day) 40.5–45 kg: 0.3 mg/day (300 mcg/day) >45 kg: 0.4 mg/day (400 mcg/day)
Clonidine ER	6 years and older: 0.1 mg (100 mcg) at bedtime	6 years and older: 0.1 mg/day (100 mcg) increments every 7 days until desired response; administered in 2 divided doses	6 years and older: 0.2 mg (200 mcg) twice daily

Abbreviations: ER, extended release; IR, immediate release.

[a] Lexidrug. Guanfacine: drug information. Retrieved March 27, 2026. https://online.lexi.com.

[b] Lexidrug. Clonidine: drug information. Retrieved March 27, 2026. https://online.lexi.com.

It is important to note that the dosing is 1 mg guanfacine equals 0.1 mg clonidine, so caution should be taken when converting doses between these medications. Similarly, the preparation of clonidine may list dosing in milligrams or micrograms depending on compounding, so the dose should be carefully verified to ensure errors are not made.

If the patient's symptoms of aggression do not improve despite adding an α_2-adrenergic agonist, consider assessing the patient's safety and the safety of caregivers and other family members in the home. Caregivers should be encouraged to seek a higher level of care if the child or adolescent displays severe aggression and is physically injuring themselves or others (eg, head banging, lacerations, burns), if there are threats of violence, or if they attempt suicide.[31,32] Cursing, stealing, throwing tantrums, skipping class, having authority issues, and damaging property are not signs of severe aggression.[31]

Partner closely with the family to provide psychoeducation, collaboratively assess stressors or triggers, refer for behavioral therapy or to community resources, and ensure feasibility of the treatment plan.[2,11] Aggression is a common reason for referral to child psychiatrists, especially when patients have had poor treatment outcomes or are taking multiple medications.[2,11] Standardized measures for aggression can help the clinician determine severity, although these are not generally used by primary care clinicians.[31,32]

- Modified Overt Aggression Scale (MOAS)
- Nisonger Child Behavior Rating Form (NCBRF)

Keep in Mind: Think Beyond Mental Health Diagnoses for Aggression Causes

- Sleep disturbance
- Food insecurity
- Bereavement
- Bullying
- Anxiety
- Trauma or abuse

Treatment for Aggression

First, treat the underlying disorder (ie, ADHD) and screen for coexisting disorders that have symptoms of aggression so these can be treated if present.[2] Next, expert consensus, including the American Academy of Pediatrics 2019 guidelines, support the use of parent education, psychoeducation, and behavioral therapy, before any pharmacological intervention.[2,31,32] Finally, if severe aggression persists, treatment with an antipsychotic may be warranted.[31–33]

Psychoeducation for Aggression

- Psychotherapy is the first line of evidence-based treatment for aggression.[31,32]
  - Specifically, behavioral therapy
- In most cases, aggression is often a behavior that is masking either an unmet need or difficulty with emotion regulation.
  - Remain nonjudgmental.
- Daily positive joint activities with parents.
  - Provide positive reinforcement.
- Focus on prevention.
  - Manage the environment.
- Promote calmness.
  - Set realistic expectations and be clear.
  - Avoid arguments.

Evidence-based parenting programs[11,13,14]

- Positive Parenting Program (Triple P)
- Behavioral Parent Training/Parent Management Training (BPT/PMT)
- Parent-Child Interaction Therapy (PCIT)
- Child-Parent Psychotherapy (CPP)

Psychopharmacology for Aggression

There are many second-generation antipsychotics used to treat aggression, but the 2 with the most evidence for the pediatric population are risperidone and aripiprazole.[31,32,34] The FDA has no approved indications for aggression in children other than irritability in children on the autism spectrum.[32] Psychopharmacology for aggression should be managed by a specialist, such as from neurology, psychiatry, or developmental behavioral pediatrics.

Integrative Therapies for ADHD

There is currently not enough evidence to support the use of complementary or integrative therapies for the primary management of ADHD.[2,33,35] However, there are some complementary practices that may be used to augment traditional care, including healthy nutrition, exercise, sleep, outdoor time, and healthy screen time limits.

Some complementary and integrative therapies with limited evidence that warrant further research and may need specialist consultation before using include[2,33,35]

- Feingold diet: elimination diet that avoids artificial food colors, flavorings, sweeteners, preservatives, and some salicylates
- Polyunsaturated fatty acids (PUFAs): supplementing with omega-3 PUFA and sometimes also omega-6 PUFA
- Vitamin D
- Magnesium
- EndeavorRx game: FDA approved video game
- Auricular therapy: acupuncture points on the ears

Caregivers should not use coffee or other forms of caffeine as a method to treat ADHD symptoms. Even though caffeine is a stimulant, it works differently and demonstrates only temporary effects on attention. For children and adolescents, the negative effects of using caffeine to treat ADHD symptoms (eg, sleep disruption, increased heart rate, potential for irritability and anxiety, and tolerance) far outweigh the minimal short-term effects.[2,25]

Follow-Up

Patients need more frequent follow-up during the initiation phase of medication and during dosage adjustments. As they reach a period of stability, visits can be spread out. The interval for follow-up needs to be personalized to the patient and severity of symptoms, as well as whether they are receiving behavioral interventions. Follow-ups may include some in-person, telephone, telehealth, or school nurse assessments, based on the patient and access to care. General guidelines include[2,25]

- Initial/acute phase
  - Every 2 to 4 weeks; visits can be telephone or telehealth visits.
  - In-person visit in 3 months to monitor growth and cardiovascular parameters.
- Active monitoring phase when the patient's condition is stable
  - Every 3 to 6 months.
  - Consider adding a visit during times of school transition or challenges, such as back to school, exams, and SATs.

Follow-up visits should include not only monitoring for symptom control, adverse effects, and growth and cardiovascular parameters but also repeating screening tools, such as the NICHQ Vanderbilt Assessment Scale. The clinician should consider using the follow-up Vanderbilt scales, especially if symptoms are not well managed or they are considering stopping medication.[2,6]

➤ If a patient started taking a stimulant at age 8 years and has been doing great, do they still need it at age 14 years?

While ADHD is a chronic condition and symptoms may persist throughout the person's lifetime, they may manifest differently at different ages. As children age and/or develop skills in psychotherapy, they often gain the ability and skills to manage their symptoms better, which may lessen the need for medication. Also, the provision of school accommodations and/or presence of supportive caregivers may make medications less necessary for adolescents.[2,11] It is important to get the patient's perspective on symptoms, side effects, and functioning to both get buy-in for treatment and help determine if stopping medication is appropriate.

If considering stopping medication, the following approach is suggested:

- Give a trial off medication on low-risk days (avoid highly academic periods including testing), such as weekends, and monitor symptoms.
- Have a teacher and a parent complete the follow-up Vanderbilt scales to compare current with previous scores.
- Discuss with adolescent patients ways in which ADHD symptoms might interfere with functioning that are unique to adolescence, such as inattention while driving, decreased functioning at work, health-risk behaviors (eg, using drugs or alcohol, having condomless sex), difficulty planning for the future or adhering to deadlines (eg, college applications), or difficulty maintaining friendships. Adolescents and their caregivers should monitor their functioning in the relevant domains and consider whether medication would help.
- Remember that a medication can always be restarted.

When to Refer

The clinician should consider referring the patient to a developmental and behavioral pediatrician, psychiatrist, and/or behavioral specialist in the following circumstances:

- Anytime they are uncomfortable with the management of the patient's ADHD or coexisting conditions
- Significant interference with functioning, including symptoms that threaten the ability to achieve developmental goals (ie, attending school)
- Treatment failure, or failure to improve after 2 medications
- Uncertain diagnosis
- Severe symptoms in children younger than 6 years
- Onset of symptoms after age 12 years
- Unusual medication side effects
- Polypharmacy complicating the treatment plan, either through drug interactions or medication side effect profiles
- Multiple mental health coexisting conditions or a concern for psychosis

Most states now have a telephonic psychiatric consultative service or child psychiatry access program that can be used by primary care clinicians for consultation, care coordination, and/or education and training programs (www.nncpap.org). Clinicians should become familiar with state-based resources. Examples of these resources include

- Massachusetts Child Psychiatry Access Project
- Commonwealth of Pennsylvania Telephonic Psychiatric Consultation Service Program
- California Child and Adolescent Mental Health Access Portal
- Virginia Mental Health Access Program

Lessons Learned About ADHD Management and Initial Treatment

Attention-deficit/hyperactivity disorder is common in children and adolescents, and management involves a combination of psychotherapy and, if indicated, psychopharmacology.[2,4,5] Treatment of ADHD can often be managed by a pediatric clinician with referral to a psychiatrist, neurologist, or developmental behavioral pediatrician only in atypical or complicated cases.[2]

- Family behavior therapy, including BPT/PMT, Triple P, and PCIT, is an evidence-based treatment of moderate to severe ADHD.[11,13,14]
- Combination therapy, with behavioral therapy and psychopharmacology, is important in the initial management of ADHD.[2,16,17]
- Stimulants are the first-line medication for ADHD.[2,24,25]
- Adverse effect management can help improve medication adherence and outcomes.[2,25]
- Review the black box warning for stimulants on the risk for diversion and misuse.[26]
- Avoid polypharmacy if possible.
- Use the validated screening tools to monitor symptoms and treatment response.[2,6]
- Reassess the treatment plan as patients age.
- Aggression may reflect poorly managed ADHD, coexisting conditions, or trauma-related dysregulation.[2,34]
- Psychoeducation and behavioral therapy should be prioritized before pharmacological interventions for aggression, emphasizing safety, emotion regulation, and relational support.[2,31,34]

Keywords: ADHD, aggression, α_2-adrenergic agonists, antipsychotics, integrative medicine, PCIT, SNRIs, stimulants

Suggested Reading

Children and Adults with Attention-Deficit/Hyperactivity Disorder (CHADD). Clinical practice guidelines. Accessed March 23, 2026. https://chadd.org/for-professionals/clinical-practice-guidelines

Danielson ML, Claussen AH, Bitsko RH, et al. ADHD prevalence among U.S. children and adolescents in 2022: diagnosis, severity, co-occurring disorders, and treatment. *J Clin Child Adolesc Psychol.* 2024;53(3):343–360 PMID: 38778436

Jensen PS. Introduction—ADHD comorbidity and treatment outcomes in the MTA. *J Am Acad Child Adolesc Psychiatry.* 2001;40(2):134–136 PMID: 11211362

Lockwood K; Children's Hospital of Philadelphia. *Primary Care Perspectives.* ADHD medication management. June 13, 2023. Accessed February 20, 2026. https://www.podbean.com/media/share/pb-ssbjk-1544c61

National Center for Health Statistics. Attention deficit hyperactivity disorder (ADHD). FastStats. Reviewed January 12, 2026. Accessed February 20, 2026. https://www.cdc.gov/nchs/fastats/adhd.htm

References

1. Weitzman C, Guevara J, Curtin M, Macias M; American Academy of Pediatrics Section on Developmental and Behavioral Pediatrics, Council on Early Childhood, and Committee on Psychosocial Aspects of Child and Family Health; Society for Developmental and Behavioral Pediatrics. Promoting optimal development: screening for mental health, emotional, and behavioral problems: clinical report. *Pediatrics.* 2025;156(3):e2025073172 PMID: 40850690
2. Wolraich ML, Hagan JF Jr, Allan C, et al; American Academy of Pediatrics Subcommittee on Children and Adolescents With Attention-Deficit/Hyperactive Disorder. Clinical practice guideline for the diagnosis, evaluation, and treatment of attention-deficit/hyperactivity disorder in children and adolescents. *Pediatrics.* 2019;144(4):e20192528 PMID: 31570648
3. Foy JM, Green CM, Earls MF; American Academy of Pediatrics Committee on Psychosocial Aspects of Child and Family Health, and Mental Health Leadership Work Group. Mental health competencies for pediatric practice. *Pediatrics.* 2019;144(5):e20192757 PMID: 31636143
4. American Psychiatric Association. Neurodevelopmental disorders. In: *Diagnostic and Statistical Manual of Mental Disorders.* 5th ed, text rev. American Psychiatric Association Publishing; 2022:68–75
5. World Health Organization. *Clinical Descriptions and Diagnostic Requirements for* ICD-11 *Mental, Behavioural and Neurodevelopmental Disorders.* World Health Organization; 2024
6. National Initiative for Children's Healthcare Quality. *NICHQ Vanderbilt Assessment Scales.* National Institute for Children's Health Quality; 2002
7. Mowlem FD, Rosenqvist MA, Martin J, Lichtenstein P, Asherson P, Larsson H. Sex differences in predicting ADHD clinical diagnosis and pharmacological treatment. *Eur Child Adolesc Psychiatry.* 2019;28(4):481–489 PMID: 30097723
8. Martin J, Langley K, Cooper M, et al. Sex differences in attention-deficit hyperactivity disorder diagnosis and clinical care: a national study of population healthcare records in Wales. *J Child Psychol Psychiatry.* 2024;65(12):1648–1658 PMID: 38864317
9. Danielson ML, Claussen AH, Bitsko RH, et al. ADHD prevalence among U.S. children and adolescents in 2022: diagnosis, severity, co-occurring disorders, and treatment. *J Clin Child Adolesc Psychol.* 2024;53(3):343–360 PMID: 38778436

10. Bitsko RH, Claussen AH, Lichstein J, et al. Mental health surveillance among children—United States, 2013–2019. *MMWR Suppl.* 2022;71(2):1–42 PMID: 35202359

11. Power TJ, Mautone JA, Soffer SL. *Family-School Success for Children with ADHD: A Guide for Intervention.* Guilford Press; 2024

12. Faraone SV, Larsson H. Genetics of attention deficit hyperactivity disorder. *Mol Psychiatry.* 2019;24(4):562–575 PMID: 29892054

13. Hornstra R, van der Oord S, Staff AI, et al. Which techniques work in Behavioral Parent Training for children with ADHD? a randomized controlled microtrial. *J Clin Child Adolesc Psychol.* 2021;50(6):888–903 PMID: 34424102

14. Phillips ST, Druskin LR, Mychailyszyn MP, Victory E, Aman E, McNeil CB. The efficacy of Parent-Child Interaction Therapy (PCIT) for youth with attention-deficit/hyperactivity disorder (ADHD): a meta-analysis. *Child Psychiatry Hum Dev.* 2025;56(6):1757–1766 PMID: 38441815

15. Vermont PBIS. Behavioral supports (students). Accessed February 23, 2026. https://www.pbisvermont.org/behavioral-supports-students

16. MTA Cooperative Group. Multimodal Treatment Study of Children with ADHD: a 14-month randomized clinical trial of treatment strategies for attention-deficit/hyperactivity disorder. *Arch Gen Psychiatry.* 1999;56(12):1073–1086 PMID: 10591283

17. Molina BSG, Hinshaw SP, Swanson JM, et al; MTA Cooperative Group. The MTA at 8 years: prospective follow-up of children treated for combined-type ADHD in a multisite study. *J Am Acad Child Adolesc Psychiatry.* 2009;48(5):484–500 PMID: 19318991

18. Children's Hospital of Philadelphia. Diagnostic considerations. Accessed April 20, 2026. https://www.chop.edu/clinical-pathway/adhd-vanderbilt-score#considerations

19. Barbaresi WJ, Campbell L, Diekroger EA, et al. Society for Developmental and Behavioral Pediatrics clinical practice guideline for the assessment and treatment of children and adolescents with complex attention-deficit/hyperactivity disorder. *J Dev Behav Pediatr.* 2020;41:S35–S57 PMID: 31996577

20. Greenhill L, Kollins S, Abikoff H, et al. Efficacy and safety of immediate-release methylphenidate treatment for preschoolers with ADHD. *J Am Acad Child Adolesc Psychiatry.* 2006;45(11):1284–1293 PMID: 17023867

21. Wigal T, Greenhill L, Chuang S, et al. Safety and tolerability of methylphenidate in preschool children with ADHD. *J Am Acad Child Adolesc Psychiatry.* 2006;45(11):1294–1303 PMID: 17028508

22. Children and Adults with Attention-Deficit/Hyperactivity Disorder. 12 behavioral programs for managing ADHD. *ADHD Weekly.* June 29, 2017. Accessed February 23, 2026. https://chadd.org/adhd-weekly/12-behavioral-programs-for-managing-adhd

23. Adesman A. ADHD Medication Guide. Accessed February 23, 2026. https://www.adhdmedicationguide.com

24. Steingard R, Taskiran S, Connor DF, Markowitz JS, Stein MA. New formulations of stimulants: an update for clinicians. *J Child Adolesc Psychopharmacol.* 2019;29(5):324–339 PMID: 31038360

25. Greenhill LL, Pliszka S, Dulcan MK, et al; American Academy of Child and Adolescent Psychiatry. Practice parameter for the use of stimulant medications in the treatment of children, adolescents, and adults. *J Am Acad Child Adolesc Psychiatry.* 2002;41(2)(suppl):26S–49S PMID: 11833633

26. US Food and Drug Administration. FDA updating warnings to improve safe use of prescription stimulants used to treat ADHD and other conditions. FDA Drug Safety Communication. May 11, 2023. Accessed February 23, 2026. https://www.fda.gov/media/168066/download

27. Faraone SV, McBurnett K, Sallee FR, Steeber J, López FA. Guanfacine extended release: a novel treatment for attention-deficit/hyperactivity disorder in children and adolescents. *Clin Ther.* 2013;35(11):1778–1793 PMID: 24139092
28. Drugs.com. Tenex: package insert / prescribing info. Accessed May 28, 2026. https://www.drugs.com/pro/tenex.html
29. Patel P, Saadabadi A. Clonidine. In *StatPearls*. StatPearls Publishing; 2026. Accessed May 28, 2026. https://www.ncbi.nlm.nih.gov/books/NBK459124
30. Pozzi M, Carnovale C, Peeters GGAM, et al. Adverse drug events related to mood and emotion in paediatric patients treated for ADHD: a meta-analysis. *J Affect Disord.* 2018;238:161–178 PMID: 29883938
31. Pappadopulos E, Rosato NS, Correll CU, et al. Experts' recommendations for treating maladaptive aggression in youth. *J Child Adolesc Psychopharmacol.* 2011;21(6):505–515 PMID: 22196314
32. Correll CU. Assessing and maximizing the safety and tolerability of antipsychotics used in the treatment of children and adolescents. *J Clin Psychiatry.* 2008;69(suppl 4):26–36 PMID: 18533766
33. Binesh M, Daghighi MR, Shirazi E, Oleson T, Hashem-Dabaghian F. Comparison of auricular therapy with sham in children with attention deficit/hyperactivity disorder: a randomized controlled trial. *J Altern Complement Med.* 2020;26(6):515–520 PMID: 32434376
34. Knapp P, Chait A, Pappadopulos E, Crystal S, Jensen PS; T-MAY Steering Group. Treatment of maladaptive aggression in youth: CERT guidelines, I: engagement, assessment, and management. *Pediatrics.* 2012;129(6):e1562–e1576 PMID: 22641762
35. Children's Hospital of Philadelphia. Alternative and complementary therapies for ADHD. Accessed April 20, 2026. https://www.chop.edu/clinical-pathway/adhd-alternative-complementary-therapies

Appendix

This table highlights selected tools discussed in the book; however, it is not intended to be exhaustive. The measures included here are evidence based; most are freely accessible to the general public, making them suitable for use in the pediatric health care setting without specialized requirements. It is important to note that additional measures exist that may involve fees and require specific training or professional qualifications to administer or interpret.

Diagnostic Concern	Tool	Description	Source
ADHD	NICHQ Vanderbilt Assessment Scale	• Screening questionnaire to diagnose and monitor ongoing ADHD symptoms, including hyperactivity, impulsivity, and inattention. • The tool is for use in children 6–12 years of age. • There are parent and teacher versions.	https://nichq.org/wp-content/uploads/2024/09/NICHQ-Vanderbilt-Assessment-Scales.pdf
Anxiety	Generalized Anxiety Disorder-7 (GAD-7)	• An efficient, 7-question self-report tool for youth aged 13–17 years for screening, diagnosis, and severity assessment of generalized anxiety disorder. • The GAD-7 does not separate types of anxiety but provides a total score. • A score of 5–9 is mild, 10–14 is moderate, and 15–21 is severe. • A score of ≥8 is considered atypical and warrants further evaluation for the presence of an anxiety disorder.	Spitzer RL, Kroenke K, Williams JBW, Löwe B. A brief measure for assessing generalized anxiety disorder: the GAD-7. *Arch Intern Med.* 2006;166(10):1092–1097 https://thereachinstitute.org/wp-content/uploads/2022/09/GAD-7_Anxiety-updated_2022.pdf
	Screen for Child Anxiety Related Emotional Disorders (SCARED)	• A pediatric anxiety screener used for children 8 years and older. • A total score of ≥25 may indicate the presence of an anxiety disorder. • Child and parent rating scale versions are available. • Additionally, this screener will give the clinician subscale scores, which may indicate a specific type of anxiety disorder such as generalized anxiety disorder, social anxiety disorder, panic, school anxiety, and separation anxiety.	Parent: https://thereachinstitute.org/wp-content/uploads/2021/06/SCARED_parent.pdf Youth: https://thereachinstitute.org/wp-content/uploads/2021/06/SCARED_child.pdf

Continued on the next page

Diagnostic Concern	Tool	Description	Source
Autism spectrum disorder	Modified Checklist for Autism in Toddlers (M-CHAT)	• A validated brief parent-report screening tool for children aged 16 months to 30 months who may be at risk for autism spectrum disorder. • If there is clinician concern after scoring, the child should be referred to a specialist for full diagnostic evaluation.	Robins DL, Fein D, Barton ML, Green JA. The Modified Checklist for Autism in Toddlers: an initial study investigating the early detection of autism and pervasive developmental disorders. *J Autism Dev Disord.* 2001;31(2):131–144
	Social Communication Questionnaire (SCQ)	• Screening tool to evaluate communication skills and social functioning in children 4 years and older who may have autism spectrum disorder. • There are 40 questions, typically completed by the parent. • It is designed to be administered by psychologists, psychiatrists, or special education teachers.	www.wpspublish.com/scq-social-communication-questionnaire.html
Behavior and/or global functioning	Children's Global Assessment Scale (CGAS)	• The CGAS is a clinician-based score of overall global psychosocial functioning on a scale of 1–100. • It is used often in research and less in clinical practice but could still give a subjective measure of overall functioning and show areas in which further assessment or intervention is warranted.	https://thereachinstitute.org/wp-content/uploads/2021/06/CGAS.pdf
	Columbia Impairment Scale (CIS)	• A 13-item tool to measure impairment in the areas of interpersonal relations, broad psychopathological domains, functioning in job or schoolwork, and use of leisure time. • For use in children and adolescents aged 9–17 years. • Parent version also available.	Parent: www.aacap.org/App_Themes/AACAP/docs/member_resources/toolbox_for_clinical_practice_and_outcomes/symptoms/CIS-P.pdf Youth: www.dhs.state.il.us/OneNetLibrary/27896/documents/By_Division/MentalHealth/Columbia/CIS-Y%20-youth%20web%20system%20version%20w%20instructions_1.pdf

Diagnostic Concern	Tool	Description	Source
Behavior and/or global functioning (*continued*)	Pediatric Symptom Checklist-17 (PSC-17)	• Parent-completed measure of a child's psychosocial functioning, normed for children and adolescents aged 4–17 years, including internalized problems (eg, anxiety, depression), attention issues, and externalizing problems (eg, disruptive and oppositional behaviors). • Consists of 17 items. • A score of ≥15 suggests the need for further follow-up and an evaluation for the presence of a mental health disorder. Similarly, each subscale has a cutoff score. — Attention—7 — Externalizing—7 — Internalizing—5 • This is a briefer version of the PSC-35.	Parent: https://thereachinstitute.org/wp-content/uploads/2021/06/psc_17_parent.pdf Youth: https://thereachinstitute.org/wp-content/uploads/2021/06/psc_17_youth.pdf
	Strengths and Difficulties Questionnaire (SDQ)	• A general behavioral screening questionnaire, normed for children and adolescents aged 2–17 years. • It focuses on emotional symptoms, conduct, hyperactivity/impulsivity, peer relationships, and prosocial behavioral concerns. • The questionnaire does not follow diagnostic criteria but can flag areas of concern and prosocial strengths. • There are 25 items; can be completed by parents, teachers, or child (age dependent).	www.sdqinfo.org

Continued on the next page

Diagnostic Concern	Tool	Description	Source
Depressive symptoms	Patient Health Questionnaire-9 Modified for Adolescents (PHQ-A)	• A depression and suicidality screening tool for youth aged 11–17 years. • The PHQ-A consists of 8 items that help classify differences in levels of depressive symptoms and 1 item related to suicidal ideation (eg, "Thoughts that you would be better off dead, or of hurting yourself in some way?"). — Cutoff scores are ▪ 5—mild ▪ 10—moderate ▪ 15—moderately severe ▪ 20—severe • If suicidal ideation is endorsed, it requires immediate follow-up with a more investigative suicide screener, such as the Ask Suicide-Screening Questions (ASQ) or Columbia-Suicide Severity Rating Scale (C-SSRS); safety planning; and referral for external support.	www.nimh.nih.gov/research/research-conducted-at-nimh/asq-toolkit-materials/asq-tool/phq-9-modified-for-adolescents-phq-a
OCD	Children's Obsessional Compulsive Inventory-Revised-Self Report) (ChOCI-R-S)	• A self-report questionnaire to assess the presence and severity of obsessive-compulsive symptoms in children and adolescents aged 7–17 years, including washing, checking, ordering, obsession, hoarding, and neutralizing.	Foa EB, Coles ME, Huppert JD, Pasupuleti RV, Franklin ME, March J. Development and validation of a child version of the Obsessive Compulsive Inventory. *Behav Ther.* 2010;41(1):121–132
	Children's Yale-Brown Obsessive-Compulsive Scale (CYBOCS)	• A clinician-administered, semi-structured interview used to assess for the presence and severity of obsessive-compulsive symptoms in children and adolescents aged 6–17 years. • It generates separate and total severity scores.	Scahill L, Riddle MA, McSwiggin-Hardin M, et al. Children's Yale-Brown Obsessive Compulsive Scale: reliability and validity. *J Am Acad Child Adolesc Psychiatry.* 1997;36(6):844–852

Diagnostic Concern	Tool	Description	Source
Safety planning	Stanley-Brown Safety Plan	• Helps identify warning signs/triggers, coping signs, and safe plans for suicidal thoughts and behaviors. • Consists of 6 topics with fill-in-the-blank sections for answers.	https://thereachinstitute.org/wp-content/uploads/2022/09/Brown-Safety-Planning-Template.pdf
Substance use	Alcohol Use Disorders Identification Test (AUDIT)	• A 10-item screening tool that assesses for risk of substance use issues including alcohol consumption, drinking behaviors, and alcohol-related problems for adolescents and adults.	https://auditscreen.org
	Brief Screener for Tobacco, Alcohol, and other Drugs (BSTAD)	• A brief screening tool used to identify substance use risk among adolescents aged 12–17. • The questionnaire assesses the number of days in the past year where substances were used, including tobacco/nicotine, alcohol, marijuana, and other drugs.	https://nida.nih.gov/bstad
	CRAFFT (Car, Relax, Alone, Forget, Family/Friends, Trouble)	• A tool for adolescents and young adults aged 12–21 that assesses alcohol- and drug-related risk behaviors. • Consists of a 9-item questionnaire and interview section.	https://crafft.org
	National Institute on Alcohol Abuse and Alcoholism (NIAAA) Alcohol Screening and Brief Intervention for Youth	• A 2-item validated, brief screening tool for youth aged 9–18 that assesses alcohol use and peer drinking behaviors in the past year. • The scale is used to identify risk for alcohol-related problems and guidance for intervention.	www.niaaa.nih.gov/alcohols-effects-health/professional-education-materials/alcohol-screening-and-brief-intervention-youth-practitioners-guide
	Screening to Brief Intervention (S2BI)	• A 7-item evidence-based, brief screening tool used to identify substance use risk among adolescents aged 12–17.	https://nida.nih.gov/s2bi

Continued on the next page

Diagnostic Concern	Tool	Description	Source
Suicidal ideation	Ask Suicide-Screening Questions (ASQ)	• Suicide risk screening tool; validated for youth 10 years and older but can be used for children as young as 8 years. • There are 4 questions; a response of "Yes" to at least 1 question is identified as a suicide risk.	www.nimh.nih.gov/research/research-conducted-at-nimh/asq-toolkit-materials
	Columbia-Sucide Severity Rating Scale (C-SSRS)	• An evidence-based screening tool used to evaluate suicide risk, including severity, immediacy, and suicidal behavior.	https://cssrs.columbia.edu/wp-content/uploads/C-SSRS-1-14-09-SinceLastVisit_AU5.1_eng-USori-1.pdf
Trauma	Child PTSD Symptom Scale for *DSM-5* (CPSS-5)	• A 27-item screening tool used to assess PTSD symptoms, severity, and impairment in children and adolescents, aged 8–18 years. • The scale has an interview version (CPSS-5-I), which takes approximately 30 minutes to complete and should be administered by a clinician or therapist, and a self-report version, which takes approximately 10 minutes to complete.	Foa EB, Johnson KM, Feeny NC, Treadwell KRH. The Child PTSD Symptom Scale: preliminary examination of its psychometric properties. *J Clin Child Psychol.* 2001;30(3):376–384 https://istss.org/clinical-resources/child-adolescent-trauma-assessments/child-and-adolescent-trauma-screen/child-ptsd-symptom-scale-for-dsm-5
	Child Trauma Screen (CTS)	• A brief 10-item screening tool that measures trauma exposure and PTSD symptoms for children and adolescents, aged 6–17 years. • Can by administered by clinical and nonclinical staff; self-report and caregiver-report versions are available.	Lang JM, Connell CM. Development and validation of a brief trauma screening measure for children: The Child Trauma Screen. *Psychol Trauma.* 2017;9(3):390-398 www.chdi.org/our-work/evidence-based-practices/screening/child-trauma-screen

Abbreviations: ADHD, attention-deficit/hyperactivity disorder; NICHQ, National Institute for Children's Health Quality; OCD, obsessive-compulsive disorder; PTSD, post-traumatic stress disorder.

Index

Page numbers followed by *f* indicate a figure; by *t*, a table; and by *b*, a box.

P